Colonialism, Catholicism, and Contraception

Colonialism, Catholicism, and Contraception

A History of Birth Control in Puerto Rico

Annette B. Ramírez de Arellano
and *Conrad Seipp*

The University of North Carolina Press   *Chapel Hill and London*

To Dr. Guillermo Arbona

© 1983 The University of North Carolina Press
All rights reserved
Manufactured in the United States of America

Library of Congress Cataloging in Publication Data

Ramírez de Arellano, Annette B.
 Colonialism, Catholicism, and contraception.

 Includes bibliographical references and index.
 1. Birth control—Puerto Rico—History. 2. Birth
control—Religious aspects—Catholic Church.
3. Contraception—Puerto Rico—History. 4. Puerto
Rico—Social conditions. I. Seipp, Conrad, 1920–
II. Title.
HQ766.5.P8R35 1983   304.6'6'097295   82-13646
ISBN 0-8078-1544-6

Contents

Acknowledgments vii

Preface ix

1. Puerto Rico as a United States Colony 3
2. A Raft Adrift 16
3. "Meddling Experiments" and the New Deal 30
4. Private Initiatives and Legal Encounters 45
5. Uphill! 57
6. The "Battle of Production" 70
7. The TVA of the Tropics 82
8. Turning Off the Faucet 93
9. An Answer to the Quest? 105
10. More Technological Fixes 124
11. A Single Instance of Inconvenience 134
12. A Matter of Conscience 149
13. Out of the Closet 159
14. Unfinished Business 173

Notes 183

Index 215

Acknowledgments

This study is dedicated to Dr. Guillermo Arbona. In the past, both of us have been associated with Dr. Arbona in various activities relating to the provision of health and welfare services in Puerto Rico. For many years, Dr. Arbona has visualized an account of the introduction and diffusion of the practice of family planning in Puerto Rico; the proposal that led to the preparation of this monograph was generated by the three of us together. Dr. Arbona actively assisted in the resulting study by helping us to identify sources of information and informants and participating in some of the interviews which were undertaken.

While we have served as the chroniclers and analysts of the following history, Dr. Arbona has been personally involved in promoting family planning services as part of a comprehensive health program. Thus he has been an intimate participant in much of the history that we have recorded. We recognize, however, that his interpretation of these events may differ at many points from ours.

We are also indebted to several individuals and institutions for support during the preparation of this manuscript. Our research was funded primarily by the Commonwealth Fund of New York. A supplementary grant was made available by the Sarah B. Gamble Trust. We are very grateful to both.

In addition to published information, it was necessary to secure primary material from archival sources. These included the Clarence J. Gamble Papers at the Francis A. Countway Library of Medicine in Boston; the Margaret Sanger Papers in the Sophia Smith Collection, Smith College; the Gregory Pincus Papers at the Library of Congress; the Rockefeller Archive Center at Pocantico Hills; the National Archives in Washington, D.C.; and the Franklin D. Roosevelt Library at Hyde Park, New York. We also benefited from documents on file at the Puerto Rico Family Planning Association and the Commonwealth of Puerto Rico Department of Health.

Many informants, too numerous to mention here, kindly submitted to interviews. In addition to answering our many queries, these sources impressed upon us the scope and complexity of the subject. José Nine Curt facilitated the use of several documents that were not otherwise available. Thomas Mathews generously provided the notes he had painstakingly indexed while researching his book *Puerto Rican Politics and the New Deal*. John L. Anderson assisted in locating or retrieving documents in the National Archives in Washington, judiciously selecting those related to our topic and tracking down particular sources, often on the basis of sketchy descriptions. José L. Vázquez Calzada, professor at the University of Puerto Rico School of Public Health, provided data and expertise concerning the demographic evolution of Puerto Rico. He also read parts of the manuscript. We would also like to thank the following persons for their comments and advice on a previous draft of the manuscript: Ernie Boyd, Betsy López, Carlos Ramos, Cecil Sheps, and Tony Thomas. Marta Nieves Koplik typed and retyped several versions of each chapter. All deserve our sincere appreciation.

Preface

The people of Puerto Rico have, for better or for worse, been studied and restudied. Probably nowhere has a society been as extensively observed, enumerated, and assessed. It often appears as though the interviewer has become a permanent and accepted adjunct of the Puerto Rican household. Computer technology has been applied to the task of counting more and more of the things that collectively make up the political, socioeconomic, and cultural life of this Caribbean island. And its recent past continues to be scrutinized and subjected both to reevaluation and, as new needs arise, to reconstruction.

The chronology of events regarding the history of birth control in Puerto Rico is relatively easy to record. An account of their intended and unintended consequences is more difficult to assemble. While the results of such analysis are by no means immune to question, they are less open to disagreement than is the interpretation we have also attempted to make of the various purposes of those who became involved in one way or another in activities touching upon the "population issue" in Puerto Rico. We see such interpretation as the critical element in this historical analysis. The dissemination and acceptance of family planning practices in Puerto Rico, as in any other society, can be understood only within the particular socioeconomic, political, and cultural history of the people.

It has never been possible to separate the promotion of family planning in Puerto Rico from "the population issue," and that issue, in turn, has reflected, refracted, and magnified virtually every other issue that has preoccupied the life of this society. It is a peculiar lens, for it often distorts and obfuscates those other issues, creating contradictory, if not illusionary, conclusions. Many of the most profound social tensions, antagonisms, and fears are expressed in it. Various segments of the society have appropriated it as a vehicle to articulate their expectations and aspirations, while it has been a shaping influence on them and those same hopes. Those who will feel impatience with the amount of attention we have given to summarizing the political and socioeconomic setting of the island and the pervasive and often drastic structural changes that have occurred in Puerto Rico in the last half century must appreciate why we feel this emphasis to be so essential. Our analysis of family planning activities in Puerto Rico hinges upon the accuracy of our interpretation of the social history of the island.

Intent is never easy to reconstruct. To capture a particular time after that present has been contaminated by subsequent events may be an impossible task. Even the most pristine memories of the participants in events have become clouded. This endeavor to explain the history of family planning in Puerto Rico is especially difficult, given the different purposes family planning has been called upon to fulfill. It has been seen as: (1) an important public health measure, for the spacing of births directly contributes to the physical, mental, and social health and well-being of both the mother and her offspring; (2) a eugenic control, protecting the genetic pool that each generation passes on to the next; (3) an instrument to catalyze economic growth and promote political stability; (4) a necessary measure to adjust to the limits of the natural environment and preserve the ecological relationships upon which human life depends; (5) a means to enable couples to engage in sexual intercourse without fear of pregnancy; and (6) a way of attaining greater equality between the sexes.

The six concerns identified here are advanced not as a basis for definitively describing the reality of the past or the present but as a crude analytical device. No particular action which is dealt with in the subsequent analysis fits completely under any one of these rubrics. Participants with various motivations combined in complex alliances to effect their desired ends. This is a recurring theme in the following account.

Another important consideration in this history is the level of the commitment of those who became involved in one way or another with "the population issue" and family planning in Puerto Rico. For many Puerto Ricans, as well as for most of the outsiders who participated in the events summarized in these chapters, family planning was a public issue which took precedence over other concerns. The intensity of their feelings for this subject is almost without parallel. For many of its proponents, it was an overriding cause pursued with evangelical zeal. Its opponents often manifested equal fervor. Accordingly, attention needs to be given not just to agreements and disagreements but to the often exceptionally passionate convictions that they engendered.

Few can be neutral about family planning; personal judgments and beliefs can hardly be excluded from a meaningful account of what actually occurred. We have attempted to capture a social reality which is part of the past and therefore presumably immutable; we want to be judged on the basis of the accuracy of our account and of the understanding that it offers. However, we do not subscribe to a positivist faith which professes the possibility of separating the world of facts from the world of values. The discriminations that are made in identifying facts must be recognized as value-laden. Facts do not speak for themselves. The validity of our analysis hinges upon our assessment of past events and how we have pieced them together into a meaningful account of what actually occurred.

Rejecting any pretense of neutrality, we must acknowledge our own value premises embedded in the historical reconstruction we have attempted. We prefer to assert these beliefs as succinctly as possible, rather than leave the reader to speculate on them. Our personal convictions concerning family planning include the following:

1. That every child born into this world has a right to be wanted.
2. That women should be able to avoid enforced motherhood.
3. That state coercion in matters regarding procreation entails an infringement on the rights of an individual.
4. That while it has become inevitable that private groups and governments should promote policies that affect procreation, there is nothing inherently commendable or deplorable about such policies. Whether population policies are progressive or reactionary depends upon the socioeconomic and political context in which they are promulgated and the way in which they are implemented; it follows that the evaluation of measures to promote family planning cannot be divorced from an evaluation of the social context in which such activities take place.

The history of family planning in Puerto Rico has intrinsic interest. It is an extensive history, stretching over more than half a century, and it unfolded in a very special setting. Because Puerto Rico is a predominantly Catholic country, the changing relations between church and state have been an important consideration. Given the island's high population density, limited natural resources, and rapid demographic growth, the question of the relation of people to resources has also been paramount. For half a century it has not been possible to consider a policy regarding family planning on the island apart from the "population problem." Thus the history of family planning is also a window for assessing and evaluating this society today, as well as for contemplating its future prospects and potential.

Both the complexity of the subject and the time span covered have conditioned the organization of this monograph. The need to consider the many events and vignettes that have occurred in the population field within their contextual framework has yielded a presentation in which background information and analysis alternate with narrative. While we have generally tried to follow a historical sequence, strict adherence to chronology would in some cases have prevented an in-depth consideration of particular issues and incidents. The three strands of colonialism, Catholicism, and contraception are thus woven into a background of profound social change which includes shifting values, industrialization, mass emigration, and technological innovation.

Colonialism, Catholicism, and Contraception

1. Puerto Rico as a United States Colony

It was manifest destiny which led the United States to acquire Puerto Rico as a territorial possession. Puerto Rico was to the United States hardly more than a minor episode in the Spanish-American War; to its inhabitants, however, the American conquest of the island was of overwhelming significance and gave rise to problems that are far from resolved today, more than eight decades later.

Early in the summer of 1898 the United States armed forces had already succeeded in crushing the military and naval power of the Spanish crown in Cuba. The scope of the conflict was enlarged in July of that year, when a large American military force landed on the southern coast of Puerto Rico. Although the American invasion was expected by the Spanish authorities, they had been led to believe that the island would be attacked from the northeast. Accordingly, the first contingents of the American army were met by only eleven soldiers of the local Spanish garrison. In occupying the island, the United States forces encountered little military opposition; in fact, they were welcomed by many. The military campaign was notable in its brevity; it lasted but seventeen days. It was also comparatively benign for both the invaders and the invaded. Total American military casualties amounted to seven killed and eighteen wounded.[1]

The Treaty of Paris, which concluded the Spanish-American War, was signed toward the end of 1898 and ratified by the U.S. Congress several months later. Among its provisions, it ceded Puerto Rico to the United States. What this country was to do with its newly acquired possession was, however, then at best unclear. Lacking in experience and uncertain in intent, the United States lapsed for twenty-five years into a policy which has aptly been characterized as "the imperialism of neglect," entailing a "policy of no policy."[2]

Often spoken of as "the gem of the Antilles," Puerto Rico had long been coveted by some Americans as a strategic outpost. With the projected construction of an isthmian canal, its military significance was enhanced. The geopolitical idea of Puerto Rico as "the Gibraltar of the Caribbean" not only commanded influence at the turn of the century, but has persisted to the present day. Thus, large tracts of the island are still the property of the United States armed forces; Puerto Rico has served as a site for army, naval, and air force installations and for missile tracking stations, as well as for a training ground at which Peace Corps volunteers are acclimatized to the indigenous conditions of the countries in which they are to serve.

Most Americans remained ignorant about Puerto Rico during the first half of this century. At best, it has been essentially taken for granted, never commanding more than the marginal attention of the political leaders in the United States. Some Americans have viewed their government's involvement in Puerto Rico as an embarrassing instance of adventurism. Increasingly, others have come to perceive the island as constituting an excessive and unjustified drain upon the American treasury. Most, however, appear to retain the idea of Puerto Rico as having some kind of strategic, political, and economic importance for the United States. The history of Puerto Rico during the last eighty years is an almost inadvertent by-product of the new national role that the United States has assumed and the emergence of new views about hemispheric and even global strategy. The expansion of American commercial and financial interests has exercised a decisive influence in defining the options open to the Puerto Rican people.

The American forces that occupied Puerto Rico in 1898 found themselves in possession of a small rectangular-shaped island hardly more than one hundred miles long and thirty-five miles wide. Behind its beaches was a littoral fringe of alluvial land, which in most places rapidly gave way to the foothills of a mountainous spine that ran its entire length. The island was endowed with great natural beauty, a profusion of tropical growth, and an equable climate. Even within the island's relatively narrow limits, however, contrasting environments could be found. On the northeastern slopes of one of its highest mountains, in excess of three thousand feet, a tropical rain forest thrived, while at its southwestern corner, desert conditions prevailed.

Despite its beauty, Puerto Rico was endowed with limited natural wealth. No mineral resources of major economic significance were known to exist.[3] The potentially valuable timbers of its forested areas had been cleared. The waters surrounding the island were restricted in their capacity to produce fish and other seafood that could be easily harvested. The economy of Puerto Rico depended upon only one natural resource, its limited supply of arable land, about half of which was then under cultivation.

Puerto Rico's agricultural development had been seriously distorted by its status as a Spanish colony. Except for a few commodities, such as ginger and hides, agricultural production was largely oriented to local needs. The larger landowners, however, amassed wealth through production for the overseas market. Trade opportunities were determined in large part by the tariffs and customs duties that the Spanish crown imposed upon that trade. Production for the overseas market became increasingly important after 1804, when Puerto Rico was allowed to trade legally with countries other than Spain. Once the door to foreign commerce was opened, Puerto Rico established an expanding network of trade relationships with other European countries, as well as with the United States and many of the islands of the Caribbean.

In 1898 coffee was Puerto Rico's most important export, exceeding in value the combined total of all others. Sugar was a poor second and tobacco a still more distant third. Only about one-fourth of its exports went to Spain.[4] By this time the Puerto Rican economy had already become dependent upon the import not only of manufactured products but also of foodstuffs. The latter, chiefly rice, wheat flour, and hog products, accounted for about two-fifths of its imports.

In 1800 the population of the island had been 150,000. With the expansion of agricultural production for overseas trade during the nineteenth century, the population increased rapidly, numbering close to 500,000 by 1850. The rate of increase slackened during the second half of the century, reaching a total of about 900,000 at the time of the American occupation.[5]

Export-oriented agricultural production arose with the introduction of slaves from Africa in the eighteenth century. However, slaves never constituted more than 12 percent of the island's population. When slavery was abolished in Puerto Rico in 1873, they numbered fewer than thirty thousand, about 4 percent of the total population.[6] Nonetheless, the practice of slavery had facilitated the expansion of the scale of agricultural production by the large landowners. Following the abolition of slavery the number of *haciendas* on the island increased. At the turn of the century there were many hundreds of sugar cane *haciendas* distributed around the island's coastal lowlands and ten times as many coffee and tobacco *fincas*, or farms, in the highlands. As many as 250 landowners cultivating cane continued to rely on their own often antiquated and inefficient mills to produce sugar. Others delivered their cane to one of the island's twenty-two major refineries, or *centrales*, to be converted into sugar. The *central* charged them a fixed percentage of the final product.[7]

Puerto Rico's overseas trade was sufficiently profitable to support a limited segment of the population in comparative affluence. The island had developed not only its own cultural tradition but a local elite that was in most respects already cosmopolitan. At the turn of the century, however, Puerto Rico's urban population was extremely small. Ponce, on the southern coast, numbered fifty-five thousand inhabitants, while San Juan, the capital, had twelve thousand less. Only three other towns had populations in excess of thirty thousand.[8] The rural population was highly dispersed in a distinctive settlement pattern. Although the landless agricultural laborers tended to live close to each other in the coastal areas, housing in the mountainous interior was often scattered on steep hillsides with limited access to the very inadequate roads. Houses in both settings were usually flimsy and overcrowded. Very few were of masonry construction, and not too many more were of wood; the majority were made of palm fronds and straw.

The class differentiation of the population was reinforced in complex and subtle ways by its physical diversity. However harshly the island's one hundred thousand or so native Indians may have been treated by their Spanish conquerors, traces of their genetic influence remain evident in the present population.[9] The consequences of racial mixing following the importation of slaves from Africa are even more pronounced. Yet many in all strata of Puerto Rican society retain the characteristics of pure European types.

The Americans who came to Puerto Rico at the turn of the century were clearly confused by the absence of the overt forms of racial segregation with which they were familiar in their own country. In many respects this has continued to be the case, for in Puerto Rico the issue of race has been the subject of a peculiar, self-imposed "conspiracy of silence," which the Americans, over the years, have by and large respected.[10] Although Puerto Rico may be free of the kind of racial discrimination that has marked relations between the races in the United States, race and the nuances of color have strong class associations and remain a major cause of anxiety for many segments of the population.

The Puerto Rican population reflected a mixing not only of races but of ethnic types as well. The island attracted settlers from Spain and, especially in the first half of the nineteenth century, from many other Mediterranean countries. The New World contributed French Cajun refugees from Louisiana and Haiti and others to this melting pot.

At the beginning of this century the population of Puerto Rico was exclusively Catholic.[11] Dominated by Spanish clerics, the church was simultaneously a central institution of Puerto Rican life and a remote and alien force. The observation of a chaplain of the American army of occupation that the island "was a Catholic country without religion whatever" was unquestionably a gross exaggeration.[12] Yet to an important extent Puerto Rico was then, as it remains today, a Catholic society in a cultural sense only.

The family was the key social unit. The position of the father as the authoritarian master within the family was reinforced by the belief in the inferiority of women. The twin ideals of virginity in unmarried women and *machismo* in men served both to enforce a profound psychological separation between the sexes and to give rise to the practices necessary to maintain different codes of behavior. This authoritarian family ideal was approximated most fully among the *jíbaros*, those living in the mountainous interior and engaged in subsistence farming and the production of tobacco and coffee. Lowlands families were more egalitarian.[13] Women within such families exercised greater freedom within the home. Differences in family structure appear to have been associated with differences in a family's relation to the land. The lowlands family, for example, was less likely than its *jíbaro* counterpart to own its own land.

At the turn of the century more than half of all Puerto Rican families were consensual unions, that is, those not officially consummated by the state. While it remains unclear whether such unions were more or less stable than marriages, consensual unions did make it easier for a woman to have children by more than one sexual partner. Thus such unions provided women with a greater measure of security by giving them entry to larger kinship networks.

Most Americans viewed the conditions that they encountered in Puerto Rico as appalling. The people were seen as dirty, ignorant, and lazy. There was a general lack of sanitation, and most families relied upon contaminated sources of water supply. Less than one-fifth of those ten years of age or over were literate.[14] Health hazards were acute, as the commanders of the American army of occupation rapidly discovered. After six months in Puerto Rico, nearly one-fourth of the troops were ineffective owing to syphilis, gonorrhea, or chancroid.[15]

Tuberculosis was rampant, a major cause of suffering and family instability as well as death. Although fewer Puerto Ricans died of malaria, its prevalence was even greater and its debilitating consequences no less devastating. Both the maternal death rate and infant mortality were at frightening levels. It is estimated that approximately one out of four newborns died during the first year of life.[16]

A member of the Army Medical Corps, Bailey Ashford, who remained in Puerto Rico throughout most of his military career, pioneered medical work to identify hookworm among the population. In 1902 he advanced the estimate that "90 percent of the rural inhabitants of Porto Rico were infested with hookworm" and that 90 percent of these "were actually sick as a consequence."[17]

Not only for infants but for adults as well diarrhea and enteritis appears to have been the leading cause of death. Widespread anemia, the combined result of chronic malnutrition and parasitic infection, seriously undermined the vitality of the society. To the Americans, the population of the island appeared lethargic and apathetic, the victims of a cultural lack of concern about time. Few apparently appreciated the extent to which the tendency toward procrastination and indifference to the present was an inevitable consequence of the population's health status.

Puerto Rico was beset with profound problems. Yet, as the end of the nineteenth century approached, many of the island's most prominent citizens felt hopeful about the future. Throughout the nineteenth century Puerto Rico, no less than Spain's other New World possessions, had been agitated by the call for independence. Puerto Rico's armed uprisings against Spain, however, had been limited and easily suppressed. Nonetheless, in the last two decades of the nineteenth century Puerto Rico had more opportunity to win concessions from Spain. As Spain lost its empire in America, Puerto Rico's strategic importance declined. This was also a period of relative economic stagnation on the island. Puerto Rico stopped attracting substantial numbers of new settlers, and Spain's domination of the island's export and import trade decreased. Puerto Rico was no longer as important to Spain as it once had been.

Ironically, a year before the Spanish-American War, Puerto Rico's leadership had successfully concluded negotiations with the Spanish crown to alter its status. The island was to be constituted as an autonomous province of Spain. Most Puerto Ricans incorrectly assumed that the United States, which existed only by virtue of its successful struggle against colonial oppression, would at least allow them to retain the degree of autonomy that they had already secured from Spain. Instead, in 1900 the U.S. Congress decreed that Puerto Rico should be maintained essentially as a ward of the American presidency. Under the terms of the Foraker Act, all basic executive and judicial authority over the island was to be exercised by a presidentially appointed governor, who would appoint his own officials. Administratively, Puerto Rico remained under the jurisdiction of the American War Department until 1934.

One of the provisions of this first law defining the relationship between Puerto Rico and the United States was the restriction of land ownership to five hundred acres or less. While this provision was motivated by a populist concern within the U.S. Congress to preserve the small farmer, the support of the sugar beet producers' lobby was crucial to its enactment. This group was interested in minimizing potential competition from Puerto Rican sugar cane. Their efforts proved to be in vain, however, because even though the five-hundred-acre limitation on land ownership was reaffirmed in subsequent legislation, no attempt was made to enforce it during the first four decades of American rule.[18]

The declaration in the Foraker Act of the American intent to incorporate Puerto Rico as an administered territory of the United States came as a shock to most of the island's leaders. With their immediate hopes for terminating Puerto Rico's status as a colony shattered, they responded in various ways. Some sought to resist what they saw as the imposition of an alien foreign master; others tried to accommodate themselves to the new arrangements; and still others attempted to win support in Washington for the provision of a greater measure of self-rule for Puerto Rico under the sovereignty of the United States. Thus were created at the beginning of this century the cleavages of political opinion that, ever since, have not only dominated the life of the island but spilled over into virtually every other area of concern.

In 1917 the U.S. Congress enacted the Jones Act, which provided the Puerto Rican people with some concessions on the form, if not the substance, of self-government. Most observers see this legislation as the consummation of a skillful and protracted lobbying campaign in Washington by one segment of Puerto Rico's elite, a campaign which coincided with the cresting of liberal sentiment in the Congress at the time the United States entered into World War I. Yet it also must be recognized as a move by Washington to check the increase of separatist political and cultural sentiment on the island by providing Puerto Ricans with a greater stake in their society's incorporation into the American union.

The most important provision of the Jones Act was the granting of U.S. citizenship to the residents of the island.[19] Although Washington retained ultimate control over the governance of the island, the Jones Act also authorized the creation of an insular bicameral legislature. It was entrusted with sufficient influence over local affairs to make party politics in Puerto Rico thereafter a major preoccupation for many, a source of income for some through either patronage or the selling of votes, and a perennially popular spectator sport for all.

The first American administrators of Puerto Rico appear noteworthy today for their ineptitude and insensitivity. Almost all reflected an exceptionally simplistic notion of what was required to accomplish what they saw as the mission assigned to them, which was nothing less than the Americanization of the population. Of marginal but emblematic importance, the spelling of the island was officially anglicized to Porto Rico, a change which persisted until 1932, when the original spelling was again formally sanctioned. More far-reaching in its consequences was the establishment of English as the language of instruction in the public school system, an innovation which required far more struggle on the part of Puerto Ricans to rescind.

Many Americans, both in and out of government, nonetheless threw themselves into the task of remaking Puerto Rican society with enthusiasm and zeal. They vigorously attacked the twin problems of ignorance and disease, made tuberculosis control and hookworm eradication the objects of comprehensive campaigns, and instituted environmental measures to sanitize the island. While some progress was achieved in reducing the disease burden of the population, those with an interest in the programs tended to make extravagant claims of success. Most of the problems were so deeply embedded in the socioeconomic and cultural circumstances of the population that their amelioration required more than the limited and individualized remedies that these efforts provided.

Later, work in the health field was further complicated when health professionals imposed the same sort of separation between preventive and curative medicine which had been institutionalized in the United States. This was done largely through the assistance that the Rockefeller Foundation provided to Puerto Rico. The creation of a public health enterprise divorced from the treatment of disease was subsequently to prove a major obstacle when the attempt was made to reorient health work as a vehicle for breaking the vicious cycle of poverty in which the society was entrapped.

Health reform was often pursued by the Americans with apparent brutality. During World War I, for example, when fifteen thousand troops were mobilized and stationed in the San Juan area, vigorous measures were taken to combat the familiar problem of venereal disease. Every known prostitute was arrested, and without benefit of trial nearly one thousand women were incarcerated for the duration of the conflict. As an American officer involved in this action observed, "Thus was a military problem met in a military manner."[20]

Although the American administrators made frequent and often colossal blunders during the first decades of this country's assumption of responsibility for the island, many of their initiatives were praiseworthy in intent. Furthermore, they often attracted dedicated recruits from the United States to assist them. Results, however, were necessarily limited, for those in positions of leadership did little to relate the attack on ignorance and disease to the need for a more general improvement in the socioeconomic conditions of the population. Few of the succession of presidentially appointed governors developed any kind of commitment to such broader reform.

Presidents treated the office as a way to reward political associates for faithful service, and those holding it acted as though they were on an extended vacation in a tropical playground. The governor who bothered to learn Spanish was the exception. All automatically restricted their involvement with Puerto Ricans to those professing loyalty to the United States. The last American who was appointed governor of the island justly made the collective characterization of his predecessors as "inept," "obtuse," "allies of the old elite," and "disinterested spectators."[21] Puerto Rico accordingly drifted in an absence of leadership.

Almost as important as the government's endeavor to Americanize the Puerto Rican population was the activity of the missionary arms of various Protestant denominations. Not only were they successful in establishing congregations in Puerto Rico but they also supported the operation of hospitals, schools, and various other community enterprises. Appealing primarily to the professional and upwardly mobile elements of the population, these churches served as important vehicles for introducing and promoting the spread of American institutions and belief systems. Following the initial success of these missions, evangelical sects began to gain influence in Puerto Rico. Those of a millennial persuasion have attracted a considerable following among the most economically disadvantaged segments of the population and, in addition, have functioned as an obscure mechanism of cultural interchange. Yet, most Puerto Ricans refused to abandon their traditional allegiance to Catholicism.

The first decades of the American rule of Puerto Rico provided many intentional and unintentional opportunities for what has been characterized as the Americanization of the population. Far more important, however, were the changes that the transfer of the ownership of the island precipitated in its economy. With the raising of the Stars and Stripes over the island, most of Puerto Rico's trade relationships were disrupted. While the new rule enhanced its access to the mainland market, it also entailed submission to the provisions of United States shipping laws and customs regulations and, ultimately, even to a quota system on the production of what was to become its most important agricultural crop. In addition, mainland interests monopolized new commercial and financial centers.

Since trade constituted such an important part of the Puerto Rican economy, such sweeping change could only have profound effects on both the character and kind of agricultural activity pursued in Puerto Rico. In addition, a devastating hurricane struck the island in 1899, inflicting such serious damage in the coffee-producing areas of the island that for the next five years output of that crop, which had been Puerto Rico's most valuable export, declined to one-tenth of what it had been before the storm.[22] Coffee production never fully recovered. This was in part because Puerto Rican traders were unable to retain their European market for that commodity. But, more important, Americans with venture capital saw the development of a sugar plantation–based economy as their most promising investment.

This entailed replacing the prevailing *hacienda* social structure with sugar cane plantations embodying capitalist relations of production. The development of an export-oriented sugar economy involved the weakening and elimination of many *haciendas* and small farms, on the one hand, and the expansion of the control exercised by a relatively few American-controlled sugar corporations on the other. By 1920 only 1.2 percent of the farms held 36 percent of the cultivated land.[23] This concentration was assisted by the government through tax laws, limitations imposed upon credit facilities, and other measures. The breakdown of the *hacienda* social organization forced the *agregados*, or tenant farmers, and small peasants either to become wage earners on the plantations or to move to the city in search of employment. By 1920 the value of Puerto Rican sugar exports was more than twice as great as the combined value of all other agricultural products. And the total volume of the island's exports exceeded by many times what it had been under Spanish rule. This, in turn, led to an increase in imports of foodstuffs and manufactured goods, and created employment in the commercial and service sectors of the economy.

Tobacco farming, concentrated in the mountainous interior, also experienced dramatic growth during the first two decades of this century. Most of this tobacco was used in the manufacture of cigars. Women represented about half the labor force in the cigar industry, although their work was confined to tobacco stripping and they were paid much less than the male cigar workers.[24] The value of both tobacco and sugar exports peaked in the early twenties, and the cigar industry declined as rapidly as it had risen.

The creation of both urban and rural working classes led to the formation of workers' unions and a workers' political party during the early years of this century. Whereas the *hacienda* social structure had fostered a culture of deference and paternalism, the expansion of the export-oriented sugar economy promoted a sharpening of class consciousness. The result of the shift from the plantation to the corporate land-and-factory combine has been described as follows: "The functions of laborer and employer are ... more sharply distinct than before—the 'employer' is corporate, and the corporate employer does not know about his laborers' lives, nor do its interests impel it to find out about them."[25]

Puerto Rico was to pay a heavy price for its increasing dependence upon the production of sugar. The collapse of the world sugar market in the mid-twenties had an immediate and devastating effect upon the island's well-being. By 1927 the average real income of Puerto Ricans had begun to decline. It continued to drop throughout the next decade as the worldwide depression exacerbated the problems of the local economy.[26] In the face of massive unemployment and widespread hunger, survival became the overriding problem for many. The Puerto Rican economy continued to provide the "after-dinner benefits" of coffee, sugar, and tobacco—"without the dinner."[27]

The steady worsening of Puerto Rico's standard of living reinforced the judgments that Americans had made about the plight of the island and its people upon their arrival at the turn of the century. With only a few notable exceptions, they had been both appalled and repelled by the conditions they encountered. "The salient characteristics of the general population ... are ignorance, poverty, and helplessness," one official wrote, expressing the general consensus.[28] At the same time they were certain in their judgment that overpopulation was a major cause of the problems they identified. Thus, in 1899, when the total population of the island still numbered less than one million persons, a military officer felt called upon to make the following observation: "The overpopulation of the island has made the struggle for existence so serious as to engender an intense selfishness, apparent in all classes of society. The poor man to whom rations have been given by the Government will sell them for rum, though his family starve. The planter who is dependent upon the peons for the labor of tilling his field seems ... to have no sense of responsibility for them."[29]

Overpopulation became a recurrent theme in all American pronouncements about Puerto Rico. When they were not indicting the people for "reckless overbreeding," they were using the presumed pressure of population upon available resources as the point of departure for recommendations for corrective actions. Thus, the American dean of the University of Puerto Rico concluded in 1917 that "the only means of meeting the situation of overpopulation is through increasing the food production of the island by means of division into small farms, intensive cultivation and modern methods of farming."[30] Yet the population then was but half as large as it was four decades later. And, as has been noted, this concern was expressed at a time when the ownership of land was becoming more concentrated and land use less diversified and the island's dependency upon imports was on the increase.

As the effects of Puerto Rico's economic stagnation became more pronounced in the later years of the twenties, alarm about the population problem mounted. Inevitably, the question of checking the rapid population growth became intertwined with issues that had at their base the political, economic, social, and cultural relationship between Puerto Rico and the United States. Neither the discussion nor the promotion of family planning in Puerto Rico could be divorced from the question of the identity of the Puerto Rican society and its relation to the United States. Family planning is obviously a personal subject and, one would think, a relatively discrete one. But this was definitely not the case in Puerto Rico. The subject of family planning, at least at the level of public discussion, could rarely be separated from its political, economic, and religious overtones

TABLE 1.1. Total Population of Puerto Rico and Selected Demographic Indicators, 1899–1930

	Total Population[a]	Rate per 1,000 *during the Previous Decade*			
		Births	Deaths	Natural Increase	Emigration
1899	953,243	–	–	–	–
1910	1,188,012	40.5	25.2	15.2	0.0
1920	1,299,809	40.4	24.0	16.4	0.8
1930	1,543,013	39.3	22.1	17.2	2.6

Source: José L. Vázquez Calzada, *La Población de Puerto Rico y su Trayectoria Histórica* (Rio Piedras: Escuela de Salud Pública, Universidad de Puerto Rico, 1978), pp. 12–14.
a. As of April 1 for each year except 1920 (January 1) and 1899 (November 1).

and implications. It thereby acted as a lightning rod for a host of more general concerns. The consideration of ways to promote the development of the society, concern about "the population problem," and support for the practice of family planning merged in a complex and rapidly changing equation.

2. A Raft Adrift

In 1922 La Democracia, *a newspaper which was the official organ of the Union* party, carried on its front page an article entitled "Practical Malthusianism," by Jacinto Ortega. The author's persuasive style and trenchant wit were less noteworthy than his identity. "Jacinto Ortega" was the pen name of Luis Muñoz Marín, the twenty-four-year-old son of Luis Muñoz Rivera, one of Puerto Rico's most prominent political leaders. Muñoz Rivera had been actively involved in Puerto Rico's negotiations to secure autonomy from Spain in the last years of the nineteenth century. He continued as a leader of the autonomist forces and had founded *La Democracia*.

Having abandoned his father's party and actively campaigned for the Socialist party in 1920, Muñoz Marín was understandably reluctant to sign the column that he sent regularly from his self-imposed exile in New York. The use of an alias provided him a forum to address his compatriots while avoiding any embarrassment to the Union party. The party leaders regarded Muñoz's articles as a way of keeping in touch with events in the metropolis while they cultivated their ties with Muñoz Rivera's heir, who showed signs of becoming a politician in his own right.[1] At the time, however, Muñoz considered himself a poet, translator, and free-lance journalist, and was contributing to a variety of publications in both the United States and Puerto Rico.[2] Writing commentaries, book reviews, and political essays, Muñoz was an avid reader who immersed himself in the literary and social currents of the day. An admirer of Anatole France and H. L. Mencken, he must have been aware of their views on population, which arose from different ideological bases but converged in their advocacy of birth control.[3] Moreover, as a member of the avant-garde living in the New York area, he was inevitably exposed to the fight for voluntary motherhood and effective birth control being waged by Margaret Sanger and others.

In his 1922 article, Muñoz declared that the ideas and methods of Sanger were necessary for the island to be "saved economically and spiritually." Although acknowledging that a better distribution of the existing wealth, an overall increase in production, and a reduction in the number of absentee owners would improve the island's economic situation, Muñoz considered these measures "too limited," preferring instead to "attack the monster [of overpopulation] by another flank." "Let us take [our island] out of poverty by reducing the number of mouths to be fed, the number of feet to be shod, the number of bodies to be clothed, the number of children to be educated. How? By following with due seriousness the doctrines held by Mrs. Sanger in the United States."[4] More specifically, Muñoz urged that the commissioner of health in each municipality be in charge of distributing contraceptives at cost to all "decent citizens" who requested them. Only thus would every child be a wanted child.

Less than a year later, in the course of an interview with a reporter from *El Mundo*, the island's leading newspaper, the young author came out from behind his pen name to declare overpopulation to be Puerto Rico's most serious problem and to repeat his solution. Describing the island as "a raft adrift with 1,300,000 victims who scratch, bite and kick to obtain the few supplies on board," he said that the grotesque circumstances in which "there is more hunger than there are meals" threatened to destroy the island's spiritual values. Addressing the imbalance between population and resources, he said:

> The problem can be attacked in two ways: reducing the population or increasing wealth. . . . I believe that reducing the population is the most important, the most practical, and the cheapest. . . . I favor Malthusianism, the voluntary limitation of childbearing, supported by the government. Scientific methods of avoiding conception should be taught to all poor families who wish to learn them, and an active campaign should be carried out so that the largest possible number of poor families will want to learn them.[5]

While Muñoz's emphasis on expediency and the poor undoubtedly reflected his belief that birth control was the solution to the prevailing economic problems, he was careful to buttress his position with a less materialistic rationale. Family planning, he argued, would have two beneficial effects: a reduction in the rate of infant mortality and the reestablishment of Puerto Rico's "ancestral cordiality and generosity." While Malthusian doctrine could be objected to on economic grounds, he concluded, "only whited sepulchres and the stupid would dare challenge it with moral arguments."

This slur upon potential opponents did not deter representatives of science and the church from entering the debate. Under the headline "The Dangers of Malthusianism" a Venezuelan physician by the name of José

Montenegro warned of the risks of upsetting the delicate balance of the endocrine glands: tinkering with the reproductive system, either artificially or naturally, would result first in neurasthenia and eventually in madness. Furthermore, he wrote, "there is no greater folly than exposing the queen of the home to such tortures, depriving her of the natural satisfaction of seeing herself surrounded by all her rosebuds."[6]

In a reply published two days later, Muñoz admitted that he was unable to counter Dr. Montenegro's scientific contentions. His "sentimental" argument, however, could be attributed only to his ignorance of Puerto Rican circumstances. "In our countryside and in our slums, children are not flowers that perfume the home, but tremendous problems that complicate the lives of our proletarians, killing their hopes and sapping their energies. Our poor families see the coming of another child to share their crust of bread as one sees the coming of a great scourge."[7]

The attack by the church was curt and did not address itself to any of the issues raised by Muñoz. Monsignor Joseph Caruana, bishop of Ponce, cataloged Malthusian doctrine as a subject which "should not so much as be named," the public discussion of such a topic being injurious to "the decorum and modesty which should distinguish Christians."[8] The bishop ended his letter by stating that Catholics committing "race suicide" would be committing an unforgivable mortal sin.

Although this declaration of Catholic dogma cut off the possibility of debate, Muñoz obviously welcomed the opportunity to further his argument in the press. In a lengthy reply published in another newspaper, he rejected the absolutist position of the church, that is, the view that certain acts are universally and unconditionally right, while others are intrinsically wrong. Instead, he advanced the relativist ethos (whereby the "goodness" or "badness" of acts is conditioned by circumstance and molded by time and place) and the teleological, utilitarian principle that holds that the morality of an action depends on its consequences.

The biblical command to "be fruitful and multiply and fill the earth," he wrote, was given when there were only two inhabitants on earth. It was not intended for India, nor for Puerto Rico. The church itself disobeyed that mandate by maintaining a celibate clergy and by allowing its followers to avoid procreation by limiting intercourse to certain periods when conception was unlikely. Muñoz described the attitude of the church as cruel, since it forced each nation to "choose between limiting the growth of its population artificially or letting nature do it brutally. A reduction in the birthrate can be achieved only by limiting conception voluntarily. The religious doctrine which condemns this procedure is also condemning humans to incalculable suffering and waste of energy."

The author then proceeded to define his concept of morality.

I see morality simply as a means to an end, and I declare my religion:
All that thwarts the development of man's highest faculties is "bad." All
that facilitates it is "good." Man's bitter competition for food and
other forms of material wealth needed for survival sharpens the lower
faculties (brute force, craftiness, dissembling) and dulls the higher ones
(reason, imagination, longing for truth). Consequently, everything that
tends to temper the fight for survival paves Nature's way to self-
knowledge through that coarse and delicate organ called Man. Hence
my neo-Malthusianism, my socialism, hence whatever Christianity
I may have.

This confession was followed by a rebuttal of Bishop Caruana's fear of "race suicide." Comparing Holland with India, Muñoz argued that unchecked population growth was more suicidal than the practice of neo-Malthusianism and proposed his goal for Puerto Rico. "My ideal is not only to assuage human suffering and economic wastefulness . . . but also to reduce population growth and even the population itself. The campaign [for birth control] in Puerto Rico would have to be more intense and persistent than that in Holland, if it is to be carried out with this objective in mind."[9]

Ending on a less serious note, Muñoz addressed himself to the prelate's threat of excommunication. This did not worry him, he indicated; he had been excommunicated since the age of eight, when his father had given him *The Three Musketeers* to read.

While Muñoz Marín's articles undoubtedly had great publicity value, his policy prescriptions were not only politically sensitive but downright illegal. In 1873 the Congress of the United States had enacted legislation that prohibited mailing, transporting, or importing "obscene, lewd, and lascivious" articles. All contraceptive devices and information were included in the ban, thereby precluding the type of intensive campaign advocated by Muñoz. These statutes were known as the "Comstock Laws," after Anthony Comstock, the founder of the Society for the Suppression of Vice and the chief promoter of moral rectitude through legislative means. In Puerto Rico, the Comstock spirit was embodied in article 268 of the criminal code, which declared the teaching of contraception a felony punishable by up to five years in prison.[10] The existing law thus had to be repealed before birth control methods could be widely disseminated and adopted.

Since article 268 had a direct bearing on the practice of medicine, it is not surprising that the law was challenged by a physician. In 1925, Dr. José

Lanauze Rolón, a Howard-trained general practitioner from Ponce, organized the Birth Control League, which had as its primary aim a change in the existing law. An avowed Communist, Lanauze admitted that his supreme ideal was "to change the entire social system from top to bottom."[11] Nevertheless, his ideology with respect to birth control had more in common with Margaret Sanger than with Marx. Whereas, in David Kennedy's analysis, Marxists generally believed that "family limitation both reduced the numerical strength of the workers, and, by alleviating their suffering, blunted their class consciousness and revolutionary fervor," less doctrinaire socialists felt that only by reducing the reserve army of the unemployed could workers hope to bid up the price of labor and obtain better living and working conditions.[12] Lanauze adopted this reformist position as a measure to bring about the "progress and happiness of the family and the community."[13]

The Birth Control League of Puerto Rico, officially founded on November 23, 1925, and including some of the leading citizens of Ponce, passed a resolution demanding the repeal of article 268 and supporting "prudential procreation" as the "first practical step towards social eugenics."[14] Birth control, the members of the league claimed, would produce healthier children, alleviate the poverty of the working class, and end the criminal practice of abortion. The failure of physicians to promote contraception, they argued, encouraged Puerto Rican women to use violent methods to terminate their pregnancies.

The league's campaign promptly received the editorial endorsement of two local newspapers, *El Mundo* and the *Times*. Both emphasized the economic and eugenic arguments in favor of reducing the birthrate of the Puerto Ricans. *El Mundo* singled out the *jíbaros* as a particular target, describing the rural population as a "generation undermined since childhood, destined, even before its birth, to pass uselessly through life, a victim of itself, of the fatal legacy left by its parents."[15] The *Times* hailed the creation of the league and attempted to preempt its potential critics. "If there are no means of getting rid of our excess population, and we must combat disease which is the only decreasing element, why not reduce our birth rate? The idea is sensible and should be encouraged even though it jars the ear of our conservative old-timers who believe in a large family whether or not they can be adequately fed and clothed."[16]

Like Muñoz Marín before him, Lanauze set forth the need for birth control in a series of newspaper articles. He also sought the help of Margaret Sanger and the American Birth Control League, with which the Ponce group wanted to affiliate itself. Sanger, desirous of co-opting "the right people" to her cause, advised him that the board of directors should represent "the best elements of the community... including a conspicuous member of the medical profession," and sent him a bibliography on birth control and samples of American Birth Control League propaganda.[17] She also referred him to the Holland Rantos Company of New York, manufacturers of pessaries, for "books and other literature."[18]

Lanauze also relied on the writings of Dr. Arletta Jacobs, Holland's first woman physician, who had opened a contraceptive clinic in Amsterdam in 1882 and introduced an improved pessary.[19] Lanauze translated Dr. Jacobs's articles into Spanish and had them published in one of the local papers.[20]

As the Birth Control League broadened its educational campaign, it inevitably provoked the opposition of the Catholic church. Two priests from the Dominican order chose to answer Dr. Lanauze's arguments, writing a series of articles in the weekly newspaper *El Piloto*.

The priests challenged Malthus's contention that population growth would outstrip available foodstuffs and advanced a number of statistics to support their point. They also argued that child rearing had a positive effect on the health of women and that later children tended to be stronger and brighter than first or second-borns. Furthermore, they felt that the fear of pregnancy served as a salutary rein on premarital and extramarital sex, thereby protecting the sanctity of marriage.

The bulk of their arguments, however, revolved around two major issues: the morality of neo-Malthusian practices and the role of sex in marriage. Concerning the former, the priests indicated that they had no quarrel with the ends of birth control; indeed, they could envision instances when family limitation was necessary and convenient and could be achieved through late marriages, celibacy, and moral restraint (as advocated by Malthus himself). The practices proposed by Dr. Lanauze, however, were intrinsically wrong and contrary to Christian morality, and had to be condemned. The ends never justify the means, they stressed, and the means in this particular case were "filthily immoral." While they considered it improper to describe the reprehensible practices in detail, they equated neo-Malthusian methods with the habit of the ancient Romans who, having feasted to the point of gluttony, regurgitated what they had eaten and proceeded to indulge their appetites once more.[21]

Dr. Lanauze rejected this analogy, indicating it was an apt description only for criminal abortion, a practice condemned and combatted by neo-Malthusians.[22] He then described the methods advocated by him as not only harmless and effective but also highly moral and dignifying because they increased marital happiness, reduced infant mortality, and provided better opportunities for life, education, and health.[23]

The second point of contention concerned the role of sex in marriage. The Dominican fathers condemned the separation of sexual intercourse from procreation, stating that the "spouses' enjoyment of carnal pleasures while artifically preventing conception" was self-indulgent and immoral.[24] To counter this argument, Lanauze advanced the "new concept of sex," that is, that sex is valuable for its own sake, regardless of its role in the production of offspring.

When appeals to reason and Christian ethics failed, each side summoned a higher authority, and each chose as an intellectual ally someone who would normally be found in the opposing camp. The priests cited George Bernard Shaw, a believer in birth control who advocated sexual abstinence as the method of choice. Not to be outdone, Lanauze contended that Jesus Christ, the "Rebel of Galilee," would have been a neo-Malthusian, even at the risk of excommunication.[25]

After almost four months of journalistic jousting the debate ended in a draw. Both sides realized that their beliefs were rooted in conflicting ideologies and that even argument was fruitless where so little common ground existed. The priests underlined the a priori existence of an absolute moral code; measured against this, neo-Malthusian methods were wrong. For Lanauze, birth control had desirable social consequences and was therefore right. In a concluding piece, the physician summed up the basic differences separating him from his adversaries. "They face the problem from the premise of an absolute, inflexible morality, ... while we study and judge it from the human point of view. ... They see in man a citizen, unhappy and tormented by his own ignorance and prejudices; we see a poor animal who has scarcely lost his tail, with a slight veneer of civilization and culture."[26]

In addition to having the last word, Dr. Lanauze delivered one final coup: when the debate was subsequently compiled and published, it was titled "The Wickedness of Too Many Children," echoing Sanger's "The Wickedness of Creating Large Families," and bore the imprint of a treatise on birth control.[27]

In his introduction to the series of articles, Dr. Lanauze asked all readers supporting neo-Malthusianism to write their legislators urging them to amend article 268. This attempt to mobilize public opinion in favor of family planning was not successful, however, and the restrictive law remained in force. The Birth Control League was disbanded around 1928, though its adherents continued to lobby for legislative changes in later years.[28] The Ponce group obtained the support of most of the local physicians and hence constituted a political force that was at least heard, if not heeded.

By the end of the decade of the twenties the majority of the Puerto Ricans were more concerned with their immediate survival than with their individual and collective futures. On September 13, 1928, Puerto Rico was hit by a hurricane, San Felipe, which left a wake of destruction as it swept from the southeast to the northwest corner of the island. The storm was responsible for over three hundred deaths; property damages were estimated at between $50 million and $80 million.[29] The island's agrarian-based economy suffered a major setback.

Sugar cane, the principal cash crop, proved to be more resilient than other products. The cane-cutting season had ended in July, and San Felipe hit during the *tiempo muerto*, or slack season. Nevertheless, the hurricane destroyed the cane stalks, and production decreased by two hundred thousand tons in 1928–29.[30] But by the following year the sugar industry had recovered, increasing its total tonnage to a level higher than previously.

Coffee, however, was dealt a more serious blow. Severely hurt by the change of sovereignty in 1898, which cost the crop its favored position in the Spanish and Cuban markets, and by the hurricane in 1899, the coffee industry had begun a painful recovery during the first decades of the twentieth century. The effects of San Felipe, however, proved devastating: coffee production dropped from 32 million pounds in 1927–28 to 5 million the following year.[31]

The damage caused by the hurricane was aggravated by the effects of the Depression, which reduced production, raised unemployment, and decreased the income of most families. As the severity of the island's economic distress increased, several studies attempted to describe the situation and prescribe measures for its solution. The most prominent of these surveys, entitled *Porto Rico and Its Problems*, was carried out by the Brookings Institution. Begun in 1928 shortly after the hurricane hit and published in 1930, the Brookings report identified Puerto Rico's rapidly increasing population as a deterrent to economic development.

> The inflow of outside capital as has come to Porto Rico would be accompanied by full employment and steadily rising standards of living. That such has not been the case . . . is primarily to be attributed to the rapid growth of population in the island. The population in 1899 was 953,243 and in 1928 it was 1,454,000, an increase of 53 per cent. The rapid growth is the combined result of an increased birth rate and a decreased death rate.[32]

The report defined the island's economic problem as that of securing the best balance between resources and productive equipment, on the one hand, and population, on the other. One of the key findings of the study was that the population had outstripped the capacity of the economy to furnish full employment and satisfactory living conditions. An array of compelling statistics was presented in support of this conclusion. Median family income was approximately $250 a year.[33] Economically productive families devoted fully 94 percent of their income to food.[34] Conditions were worse among the unemployed, who represented 27 percent of the labor force.[35]

The health conditions and patterns of illness reflected the extent and severity of poverty. The principal causes of death were diarrhea-enteritis, tuberculosis, and malaria; these accounted for more than 40 percent of all deaths. Uncinariasis, or hookworm, while not ordinarily fatal, was described as "more stealthily dangerous" because its weakening effects incapacitated its victims and made them more susceptible to other diseases.[36]

The emphasis given to rural conditions reflected Puerto Rico's population distribution and occupational structure. Rural inhabitants constituted over 72 percent of the total.[37] Moreover, more than half of the labor force was employed in agriculture, and two-thirds of the population depended on this sector for its livelihood. The report pointed out that, by U.S. standards, the island could hardly be described as a farming community; rather, it was a community of agricultural tenants who "own [neither] the land that they till nor the crops that they raise."[38] Since four out of every five families living in the country were landless, agricultural wages, crop diversification, and land tenure were fundamental matters for the island's economy. In its conclusions, however, the Brookings report skirted the issues of sugar monoculture, absentee ownership of the agricultural estates, and the concentration of landholdings into a few *latifundia* and the resultant powerlessness of the dispossessed tenant farmers.

The dependence on sugar was justified as economically rational, since production of that crop yielded the highest return. Absentee ownership on the part of the sugar corporations and the siphoning off of the island's wealth were hardly considered problems; indeed, the cosmetic remedy proposed for this particular ill was that of "increasing Puerto Rico's attractiveness as a place of residence" through the promotion of city planning, the development of restricted residential suburbs, and the provision of cultural amenities.[39]

Similarly, the concentration of land in large holdings was regarded as advantageous in financial and technical terms; changes in the system of tenure were thus deemed ineffectual and possibly undesirable. The report urged the repeal of the "futile law" limiting agricultural corporations to a maximum of five hundred acres, arguing that this law simply made the intelligent control of such enterprises more difficult.[40] In short, the Brookings study opted for efficiency over equity and concluded that no agrarian remedy was likely to solve Puerto Rico's difficulties.

With all possibilities of basic agricultural reform thereby dismissed, the report explored two further avenues: the expansion of other means of production and the control of population. Recommendations concerning the former included the development of local industries, particularly those using imported materials; the encouragement of national thrift; and the improvement of marketing facilities and methods.[41] The reduction of the population, however, was seen not only as the more promising alternative but also as a precondition for development. Emigration was considered too difficult, and thus birth control emerged as the only choice.[42] "The people of Puerto Rico . . . have bred up to—and indeed beyond—the normal subsistence line. . . . As long as this continues permanent economic betterment for the masses is impossible. Education in parental responsibility provides the only remedy."[43]

By in effect defending the island's existing socioeconomic structure and selecting population as the variable in the population-resources issue more amenable to change, the Brookings report gave respectability to the view that fertility rates could be acted upon without changing the political, social, and economic context within which demographic decisions are made.[44] Thus the advocacy of birth control by the Brookings group was a conservative measure, aimed at preserving the economic status quo and maintaining the prevailing social order.

This paradigm did not go unchallenged, however. A second study, carried out by Bailey W. and Justine Whitfield Diffie under the sponsorship of the American Fund for Public Service, described the situation in terms similar to those of the Brookings publication, but was more radical concerning what was required.[45]

The Diffies pointed out that for every square mile of food crops grown for local consumption there were "about 9,000 people who must be fed, clothed, housed, insured, doctored and educated."[46] Nevertheless, they refused to consider this the root problem of Puerto Rico's economic ills, or the main cause of unemployment. "That the population is excessive has already been shown, and there is no doubt that a decrease would serve to alleviate the widespread suffering; but the density of the population must be accepted as one of the difficulties to be met in working for better social conditions, and not merely as a lame excuse for the inactivity so far characteristic of the United States government."[47]

Unlike the Brookings report, the Diffies decried the nonenforcement of the five-hundred-acre law and the plantation economy that had grown up as a result of that nonenforcement. The figures showing rising production were deceptive, they said, giving the impression of a prosperous Puerto Rico, while

> the truth is that the majority of the people of the Island are actually being forced further into debt day by day. . . . The industry does not belong to natives, but to outsiders. The profits are not enjoyed by those who make them possible, but by those who never see Porto Rico. The wages . . . are miserably inadequate for the sustenance of life. . . . However glittering the sugar industry may appear to outsiders, the Porto Ricans know that it has not paid. "Sugar economy" has proved to be "bad economy" for Porto Rico.[48]

The Diffies' position that the island's economic imbalances and structural difficulties could not be attributed to excess population struck a responsive chord among the Puerto Rican nationalists, who, according to historian Linda Gordon, "perceived birth control as a U.S. manufactured ideology, a form of cultural imperialism, and above all a means of deflecting attention from the deepest problems of the island and a permanent solution to them."[49] In a letter to the editor of the *Birth Control Review*, founded by Margaret Sanger, J. Enamorado Cuesta, secretary of the Nationalist party, emphasized the importance of the political context within which population policies are made.

> There is no denying that overpopulation . . . is at present a problem to us. . . . It is directly at the door of American capitalism that the blame must be laid for everything that is wrong in Porto Rico today. . . . When American intervention was started, while sanitary conditions were certainly not very good, still our people owned their land, the produce they exported. . . . in thirty-four years of American intervention, . . . the people have been dispossessed of their land and brought to the condition of paupers. . . . This does not mean that I am systematically opposed to birth control. But our real problem lies in the actual control by American capital of practically all our wealth. . . . We may, and we may not, enact birth control laws (I think we would) as soon as the American flag is lowered from our public buildings.[50]

Less moderate nationalists believed that birth control was part of a genocidal plan to systematically exterminate the Puerto Rican people. This view gained unanticipated credibility from an incident involving Dr. Cornelius Rhoads, who was working in San Juan's Presbyterian Hospital under the auspices of the Rockefeller Foundation. In a chatty letter to a friend, Dr. Rhoads had revealed his hatred of the Puerto Ricans and confessed to eliminating some of them. The unmailed letter was picked up by one of his laboratory assistants, circulated among the hospital staff, and eventually published in the January 27, 1932, edition of *El Mundo*. From the text of the letter, it is easy to see why it made front-page news. Dr. Rhoads had written:

> The Porto Ricans . . . are beyond doubt the dirtiest, laziest, most degenerate and thievish race of men ever inhabiting this sphere. . . . What the island needs is not public health work but a tidal wave or something to totally exterminate the population. It might then be livable. I have done my best to further the process of extermination by killing off eight and transplanting cancer into several more. The latter has not resulted in any fatalities so far. . . . The matter of consideration for the patients' welfare plays no role here—in fact, all physicians take delight in the abuse and torture of the unfortunate subjects.[51]

Dr. Rhoads insisted that the letter was written in a fit of anger and did not reflect his true feelings or performance. The recently appointed governor, James R. Beverley, responding to the demands of the press, the medical profession, and the nationalists, ordered an investigation of the legal and medical aspects of the case to see if Dr. Rhoads could be prosecuted for libel or murder. No grounds were found for the first charge, however, since the doctor had not purposely made public his libelous statement.[52] An epidemiological investigation was unable to attribute any deaths to negligence or malpractice on the part of the physician. As a result, no formal charges where ever brought against Dr. Rhoads.[53] In fact, Dr. Rhoads went on to become the director of the Sloan-Kettering Institute in New York City. (It has subsequently been disclosed that Dr. Rhoads wrote an even more damaging letter. This second letter was effectively suppressed in the course of the investigation and has only come to light in recent years.)[54]

Although this incident arose during his first week in office, Governor Beverley, a Texas lawyer who had been in Puerto Rico since 1925, decided to approach the population issue directly. In his inaugural address on January 30, 1932, he spoke of the need for Puerto Rico to stress the quality of its population rather than the quantity and indicated that "sooner or later the question of our excessive population must be faced."[55] Privately, Beverley bemoaned the dysgenic effect of fertility differentials between classes and the possibility of civil strife brought about by the existence of "a permanently depressed population a large part of which is living on the verge of starvation."[56] Publicly, however, he expressed his support of population control as a development tool.

The governor's official report for 1932 suggested that the riches of "King Sugar" were not trickling down to the average Puerto Rican.[57] Nevertheless, it did attribute the island's economic problems to an excess number of inhabitants and indicated a decrease in population as the way out of the poverty trap.

> For the problem of overpopulation a number of partial solutions have been advocated. Up to the present time the government has given attention to the encouragement of new industries and the expansion of established ones, but it seems clear that it is rapidly becoming necessary to attempt other and further solutions. . . . The population question is fundamental and is intimately related to the standard of living, to labor conditions and especially to health conditions.[58]

The governor's mention of "other and further solutions" brought forth a storm of protest. The Reverend A. J. Willinger, bishop of Ponce, spoke out against Beverley's advocacy of birth control, and the National Catholic Alumni Federation—boasting three hundred thousand members in the United States—wrote President Hoover and Secretary of War Patrick J. Hurley demanding that Beverley publicly withdraw his statements regarding birth control and cease dealing with the topic.[59]

Even as the controversy was raging, a group of private citizens decided once again to establish a birth control league, this time in San Juan. Unlike its predecessor in Ponce, the new league intended to provide services as well as orientation. Its objectives were "to promote and propagate sexual education, especially among the poor people, relating to the medical, economic and sociological aspect of birth control; [and] to assist in financing suitable and proper Maternal Health Centers where women may receive proper advice and instruction under medical supervision for the cure and prevention of disease, so as to be able to develop strong and healthy future generations, and thus avoid the grave social problems of venereal disease and dependency."[60]

Headed by an attorney, Carlos Torres, and his wife, Estella Alcaide de Torres, the league was established as a nonprofit corporation under the laws of Puerto Rico. Government authorities immediately questioned whether the purposes of the corporation violated section 268 of the criminal code and asked the attorney general for his opinion concerning the legality of the new entity. The attorney general was obviously sympathetic to the birth control cause and chose to give a narrow interpretation to both the objectives of the league and the dispositions of the code.

> It seems that . . . the purpose [of the league] will be effectively emasculated if the corporation obeys the law, but it is possible to place a lawful interpretation upon it. Such being the case, we have no right to assume that the incorporators intend to break the law. It is possible, although verging on absurdity, that the incorporators intend to advocate continence as the most hygienic and effective mode of birth control. Such a view has been advanced by a very high authority, and is not . . . contrary to law.[61]

The attorney general therefore concluded that none of the league's objectives were unlawful per se and that the organization could not be refused a certificate of incorporation.

Once this legal skirmish had been won, there were financial and administrative obstacles to overcome.[62] But on November 21, 1932, the Birth Control League of Porto Rico opened its first clinic in San Juan and began providing contraceptive services under the direction of a physician and a registered nurse.[63] In 1933 a clinic was also opened in the town of Mayagüez.[64] Despite the blessings of Margaret Sanger and the indirect backing of the governor, these efforts were short-lived. Lack of public support, religious opposition, and a scarcity of funds finally led to the league's demise.

Nevertheless, the years between 1922 and 1932 witnessed the initiation of public discussion concerning overpopulation as a problem and birth control as a solution. The writings of Muñoz Marín and Lanauze Rolón, together with the reactions they elicited from the church and the press, represented the first sounding of many themes that were to be repeated in subsequent decades. Similarly, the official pronouncements of Governor Beverley and the Brookings Institution successfully incorporated the population question into Puerto Rico's political agenda. Programmatic endeavors in the area of family planning were therefore subject to the vagaries of political change, and services varied in relation to private promotion and public policy.

3. "Meddling Experiments" and the New Deal

Historian Arturo Morales Carrión has characterized the decade of the thirties in Puerto Rico as a period of "intense dissatisfaction, political turbulence, an anguishing analysis of the historical foundations of a country appearing to drift aimlessly, without helm or compass."[1] It was for Puerto Ricans a period of unrelieved despair, wondrous only in that it did not crush their spirit completely. Traditionally, members of the Puerto Rican laboring class had been dependent upon patrons for their welfare, but in the thirties their dependency was quite literally transferred to the remote workings of government officials in Washington.

Whatever enthusiasm greeted the election of Franklin Delano Roosevelt in the United States in 1932, that elation was scarcely felt in the colony of Puerto Rico. Except for the local Democratic party clique that started jockeying for the political patronage jobs that became available, the Puerto Rican population, suffering the effects of yet another hurricane, was too preoccupied with its own difficulties to worry or care about the repercussions that mainland policies could have on the island. Yet the new president had the power to designate the island's governor, and that decision would in turn affect the lives of Puerto Rico's more than 1,500,000 inhabitants.

As early as November 1932, President-elect Roosevelt had been advised that the governorship of the island required "a man of the highest type of intelligence and experience, . . . a man who has courage, tact, knowledge of government and politics, and a sense of humor."[2] Seeming to ignore that advice, however, he chose Robert H. Gore, later described as "one of those fantastic characters who turn up once in a while in such posts."[3] Gore had been an early supporter of Roosevelt and had contributed generously to his campaign. Thinking that being a Catholic was the only qualification for the highest public office in Puerto Rico, one of the president's political brokers recommended Gore, who met that criterion.[4]

Like his predecessor, Gore addressed the population question in his inaugural address. Unlike Beverley, however, he indicated that he was "not an advocate of the suppression of the human race by birth control." Instead, Gore proposed settling Puerto Rican families in agricultural communities in Florida, where a similar climate and rich soils would provide a hospitable environment for the immigrants.[5] Although welcomed by some of Puerto Rico's political leaders, this suggestion was roundly denounced by the president of the Nationalist party, Pedro Albizu Campos. After congratulating Gore for his rejection of birth control, Albizu rejected the governor's emigration plan, noting that "the Yankees desire the cage but not the birds."[6]

Gore espoused statehood for Puerto Rico and the Americanization of the school system, thereby antagonizing those who sought greater political autonomy and the protection of Puerto Rico's language and culture. In time, Gore's insensitivity and ineptness succeeded in alienating even his potential allies. It was rumored that the bishop of Ponce had written to his ecclesiastical superiors in the United States to protest Gore's continuation in office; the governor's presence was considered harmful to the reputation of the Roman Catholic church in Puerto Rico.[7] As the attacks on him became more frequent, varied, and strident, Gore became mired in local politics and was increasingly ineffectual.

Gore's incompetence was somewhat cushioned by the federal funds that became available under the new administration. During his campaign, Roosevelt had used the expression "New Deal" to refer to a variety of policies, programs, and proposals designed to bring about domestic reform and economic recovery. Once in power, he moved quickly to enact the legislation required for the promised New Deal. One of the agencies created in the feverish pace of the Hundred Days was the Federal Emergency Relief Administration (FERA), which provided federal funds to state and local governments for most forms of direct relief. The program was based on a cost-sharing formula, the federal government supplying one dollar for every three put up by the local government. This requirement delayed Puerto Rico's participation in the relief effort; the insular government, overextended in loans, could not put up the matching funds required to bring in the federal aid.[8]

This requirement was eventually waived, and in August 1933 the FERA selected James Bourne to direct the Puerto Rico Emergency Relief Administration (PRERA). Bourne had been a plant superintendent for the Hill Brothers canneries in Puerto Rico and had lived on the island for three years.[9] His wife, Dorothy Bourne, had organized the School of Social Work at the University of Puerto Rico and added her expertise to her husband's managerial functions. The Bournes were former residents of Hyde Park and were good friends of President Roosevelt and his wife. This facilitated communication with the chief executive and permitted the PRERA much autonomy vis-à-vis Governor Gore and the local politicians.

By fall, Gore was ruing the day on which he had accepted the governorship and complaining to an officer of the FERA that "conditions on the island are so bad that it has taken the heart completely out of me and I wish to God that I were not on the Island. . . . A land that is starving has nothing but discontentment."[10] At the same time, the Bournes were busy organizing their agency and expediting the use of PRERA funds for direct relief and work projects. James Bourne also submitted a report entitled "A Constructive Plan for Puerto Rico"; this outlined particular areas to which the PRERA should devote its attention. Suggested projects in the health field included malaria control, the construction of tuberculosis sanitaria, and the establishment of a latrine service.

In his report, Bourne stated that the problem of overpopulation was "the most serious question to be faced by any farseeing administration." In addition to emigration to nearby Spanish-speaking countries, he recommended a widespread plan for birth control.

> Intelligent and scientific control of population seems most feasible and necessary. It is a matter of education of the people and overcoming the prejudices of the Catholic Church. Birth control education could be carried on through the existing health units without increasing the personnel, providing the present law was altered (not joining birth control with abortion as a criminal offense).[11]

Despite the legal constraints, Bourne decided to incorporate birth control into the activities of the PRERA. The politics of malaria control, however, made him reconsider his initial idea of carrying out family planning through the existing health units. The PRERA had delegated the direction of its malaria control project to the Department of Health. The method used was the elimination of the breeding places of the mosquito vector by drainage or filling. In practice, this program was carried out selectively, on the properties of several of the important members of the Senate who were also leaders of the Republican party then in power. Bourne called this "perhaps legal but not ethical," and he resolved to avoid this type of incident by carrying out any public health work paid for with relief administration funds under the direct supervision of his agency.[12]

The PRERA's education division proved to be an apt vehicle for the dissemination of contraceptive information. In addition to providing resources for the understaffed public school system, this division established day-care centers, nursery schools, and a program of adult education. This last included literacy classes, vocational training, and parental education aimed at "teaching parents their responsibilities with respect to child-rearing and family life."[13] The PRERA also published a magazine, *La Rehabilitación*, which had articles on sex education and marriage and the family,[14] and stated in its *First Annual Report* that "through education and medical advice leading toward the better health of mothers and children, as well as considering the probable future under existing conditions, attempts must be made to keep the population of the Island within the possibilities of decent living."[15]

Yet, for all its efforts, the PRERA was limited to carrying out a series of stopgap measures designed to mitigate the most glaring defects of Puerto Rico's colonial economy. Its mandate was relief, which precluded its undertaking more fundamental economic reform. This was the island's major concern in March 1934, when Eleanor Roosevelt visited Puerto Rico. Coincidentally, Assistant Secretary of Agriculture Rexford Tugwell was on the same plane from Miami on a political and fact-finding mission.

During their stay the visitors toured the island and met with politicians, government officials, and representatives of the University of Puerto Rico, agriculture, commerce, industry, and the church. While still on the island, Tugwell wrote Secretary of the Interior Harold Ickes and Secretary of Agriculture Henry Wallace concerning his impressions. Although he feared the dysgenic effects of birth control, both the island's low standard of living and the possibility of a mass migration of Puerto Ricans to the United States transformed Tugwell into an advocate of family planning. To Wallace he wrote:

> The precariousness of all this seems to be realized by nature, and she compensates by an enormous fecundity. There are a dozen children behind every bush, many of them very indifferently nourished. But nature aided by our doctors has only added to the prevailing difficulty by such a growth of population that it outruns any possibility of furnishing opportunity in our terms.
> There will be something like a crisis here soon . . . with the pressures that are accumulating. There must be either an increase in our charity or a mass movement outward of population. . . . I rather dislike to think that our falling fertility must be supplemented by these people. But that

will probably happen. Our control of the tropics seems to me certain to increase immigration from here and the next wave of the lowly... succeeding the Irish, Italians, and Slavs... will be these mulatto, Indian, Spanish people from the south of us. They make poor material for social organization but you are going to have to reckon with them.[16]

Upon his return, Tugwell wrote President Roosevelt the extensive "Report on American Tropical Policy." In it, he once again stressed the "abundant and prodigious life of the tropics" and described the average Puerto Rican in terms reminiscent of Rousseau's noble savage.

Confronted with low living costs and the unabashed fertility of nature, the Puerto Ricans increase and multiply. They love children, the women are not afraid to bear them and the men have no reluctance to beget them, practicing a loose variant of polygamy for that purpose, with which the women are content. They are happy and light-hearted and, observers agree, come far closer to getting what they want out of life than most people in the United States.[17]

The belief that the "Puerto Ricans would rather have more children than increase their standard of living," Tugwell continued, called for very slow and wise action on the part of the United States.[18] Nevertheless, he proposed a two-pronged approach to improve the island's standard of living. "A fuller and more effective use of the resources must be made and a more equitable distribution obtained than is now the case. At the same time a recognition on the part of the Islanders themselves must be developed by which they will become conscious of the fact that an improved standard of living... is possible only to the extent that a definite check on the increase of population is made."[19]

In a memorandum following a meeting with the president, Tugwell once again brought up the population question in Puerto Rico. Discussing possible alternatives for a long-term reconstruction plan for the island, he made four recommendations that focused on expanding or redistributing the island's economic resources: socializing the sugar industry and operating it through a government corporation; establishing light domestic industries; promoting the growing of vegetables; and actively promoting fishing, forestry, and crops such as cotton, quinine, and rubber.[20] A fifth point involved encouraging the control of population. Although this was considered "the most difficult of many difficult problems," the memorandum urged using every channel possible "to place in every family both the knowledge and the means of preventing childbirth."[21]

Tugwell, however, was wary of imposing his suggestions or of giving the Puerto Ricans "what [he thought] they ought to want." Instead, he recommended that "Dr. Carlos Chardón, Chancellor of the University, and the Governor of Puerto Rico select a small informal committee of representative men, not more than five and preferably three, from the Island, to come to Washington and ascertain what services and facilities the Federal Government may dispose of which would be useful to Puerto Rico."[22]

Shortly afterwards, the president acted on this suggestion and the Puerto Rican Policy Commission came into being. In addition to Chardón, who chaired the group, the commission was composed of Commissioner of Agriculture Rafael Menéndez Ramos and Rafael Fernández García, a professor of chemistry at the University of Puerto Rico. Luis Muñoz Marín, who had rejoined his father's party and been elected senator in 1932, tried to get an official invitation to join the commission, but was unsuccessful. Nevertheless, he was told that he would be welcome to attend the commission's conferences.[23]

The three members of the commission spent the months of May and June 1934 in Washington, drafting their report. Muñoz Marín, eager to share the limelight and participate in the commission's deliberations, took advantage of the informal invitation extended to him and joined the group in Washington. Indeed, the plan that was presented to President Roosevelt on June 14, 1934, bore the young senator's imprint: he had drafted the introduction, which recalled the basic themes he had expounded on a decade earlier while writing as "Jacinto Ortega."[24]

The Chardón Plan, as the report of the commission came to be known, attempted to be a complete blueprint for the economic reconstruction of Puerto Rico. In its first sentence the introduction defined the economic problem of the island as "progressive landlessness, chronic unemployment, and implacable growth of the population."[25] It then went on to state the dual purposes of the plan—the restoration of the land to the people that cultivate it and the fullest development of the island's industrial possibilities—but indicated that these could not be achieved without checking or reducing population growth.

> Even if a parity between population and employment . . . can be approximately achieved, it cannot be maintained unless the rate of population growth can be kept within the scope of further economic development. It therefore seems desirable, probably imperative, that a land restoration and industrial development program, combined with a policy of emigration to suitable environment, be fully worked out as soon as possible.[26]

The choice of emigration over contraception as a means of population control was buttressed by the argument that reductions in fertility follow rather than precede economic development.

> Although a scientific scheme of birth control should be part of any farsighted policy for Puerto Rico, it cannot be hoped that it will be socially effective until the standard of living, and therefore the sense of responsibility of the mass of the population, has been substantially improved. It will probably be effective in keeping the rate of growth down in the future, after the improvement brought about by economic reconstruction has begun to be felt by the population as a whole.[27]

The type of emigration proposed was that of "mass colonization projects in under-populated regions of tropical countries similar to Puerto Rico . . . in climate . . . , language, religion, racial stock, traditions, and culture."[28] It was also contemplated that entire communities, rather than individuals or families, would emigrate, thereby avoiding social dislocation and labor exploitation. Santo Domingo, Cuba, Costa Rica, Venezuela, and Brazil were suggested as possible destinations.

The Chardón Plan, however, was primarily aimed at increasing resources rather than checking population growth. Among its objectives were: (1) increasing returns to farmers and workers from the operation of the sugar industry; (2) stemming the outflow of millions of dollars as a result of large absentee holdings; (3) preventing the disappearance of the small farmers, who were being swallowed by the large corporations; and (4) augmenting the local production of foodstuffs.[29]

These objectives were to be realized by the establishment of a corporation that would acquire productive sugar lands and operate the mills included on these lands. This corporation would operate at least one sugar mill as a "yardstick" for regulating future relationships between the *colonos*, or tenant farmers, and the mill owners. Profits in excess of 8 percent would be used for further rehabilitation work. In addition, the corporation was to exchange productive land for marginal cane lands, using these for subsistence homesteads and the production of small cash crops.[30]

Because the plan would have drastically altered the power and profits enjoyed by the sugar industry, it was attacked as soon as its recommendations became known. Although the president indicated that he had given the proposals his approval "in principle" and later stated that the Chardón Plan was to be the basis for the island's rehabilitation, no concrete action was taken with respect to agricultural reform.[31]

Instead, Washington attempted to show its concern for Puerto Rico and still bide its time by two well-known and frequently used dilatory devices.

The first was the naming of a study committee, the Inter-Departmental Committee for the Economic Rehabilitation of Puerto Rico, to "work out a coordinating plan and advise on the general rehabilitation program of Puerto Rico."[32] One of its tasks was to study the Chardón Plan in order to appraise its feasibility and coordinate the federal agencies involved in its implementation. The committee in turn named a technical committee of three persons to go to Puerto Rico and report on the problems involved in carrying out the proposed plan.

The second tactic involved a restructuring of the federal bureaucracy that dealt with Puerto Rico. Following Tugwell's advice, Puerto Rican affairs at the federal level were removed from the jurisdiction of the War Department. The Division of Territories and Island Possessions was created in the Department of the Interior to supervise federal relations with Hawaii, Alaska, the Philippines, the Virgin Islands, and Puerto Rico. During the summer of 1934, Dr. Ernest Gruening was appointed director of the new division. Because Roosevelt had characterized Puerto Rico's situation as "hopeless," Gruening understood that he should give the island priority over his other "three wards."[33]

The designation of Gruening proved to be significant in implementing a program of birth control in Puerto Rico. Trained at Harvard Medical School, Gruening had been impressed by the effects of excessive childbearing on the health of women from the slums of South Boston.[34] After graduation, he chose a career in journalism over medicine and became managing editor of the *Nation* and a crusader for birth control. When Margaret Sanger organized the First American Birth Control Conference in 1921, Dr. and Mrs. Gruening were asked to be members of the conference committee. On the third day of the conference, Sanger was arrested as she began to address the audience. According to the *New York Times*, a police raid of the meeting had been ordered by Archbishop Patrick Hayes of New York, who subsequently denounced supporters and practitioners of birth control as "worse than murderers."[35] Thinking it advisable "to balance the fulminations of Archbishop Hayes—shortly to be made Cardinal—with the views of another prominent interpreter of the divine purpose," Gruening asked the dean of St. Paul's Cathedral in London to write an article for the *Nation* on the importance of planned parenthood.[36]

In Puerto Rico, Gruening's immediate problem was to create an agency to carry out the Chardón Plan's proposals and find the means of funding them. Hopeful that the PRERA could assume the new and expanded functions of economic reconstruction outlined in the plan, Bourne continued to carry out his relief efforts with determination.

Faced with dwindling support from the federal government, Bourne was also losing political ground in Puerto Rico. The party in power, a coalition of Republicans and Socialists, charged the PRERA with favoritism toward Muñoz Marín and his party, now constituted as the Liberal party. It also chose to make political capital of the PRERA's support for birth control, knowing that this issue was potentially volatile and could galvanize the opposition of the Catholic church.

In March 1935 the legislature passed a concurrent resolution concerning Puerto Rico's social and economic problems. The resolution pondered the eugenic possibilities of birth control, but did not consider this an adequate means to solve the island's population problem. Instead the legislature favored the judicious application of scientific agricultural technology, which would increase production several fold and allow Puerto Rico to support a population of over twenty million inhabitants.[37]

In April 1935 the governing coalition sent a social worker who had worked with the PRERA to Washington to present charges concerning the agency's birth control activities before the Roman Catholic authorities.[38] After this woman, whom Bourne termed "spiteful,"[39] had described the PRERA's maternal health campaign, John J. Burke of the National Catholic Welfare Conference wrote President Roosevelt to complain that Bourne was "using the monies of the United States to violate the Penal Code of the United States in Puerto Rico. . . . Mr. Bourne is paying women workers in Puerto Rico to manufacture preventatives that are used to prevent conception. [He] is paying for the training of workers who, in turn, are advising the married women of Puerto Rico in the practice of birth control. . . . Mrs. James Bourne . . . is actively and publicly promoting birth control."[40] The letter therefore urged the president to "remove both Mr. and Mrs. Bourne for violation of the laws of the United States."[41]

The controversy escalated when the island's church hierarchy joined in the protest. Unlike their Spanish predecessors, the American bishops were conscious of their minority status and were therefore schooled in the tactics of pressure politics. Monsignor Willinger, the bishop of Ponce, wrote Dorothy Bourne to inquire about the type of contraceptive information provided by the PRERA. She answered that physician-approved advice given for proper health reasons by a member of the medical profession was being provided "to persons who have no religious scruples against receiving such information."[42]

This explanation of the methods and clientele of the PRERA program did little to calm the Catholics' fears. Catholic Action, a lay organization from Ponce, wrote President Roosevelt to request that no program promoting birth control practices be included in the rehabilitation or reconstruction plan for Puerto Rico, since such practices were "contrary to the Principles sustained by the Catholic Religion which is professed by the great majority of the people of this island."[43] Similarly, Bishop Edwin V. Byrne of San Juan urged Gruening to avoid the trouble that he would provoke by "foisting birth control in this Catholic country."[44] Gruening assured him that no such project was contemplated, since this was neither "a governmental function [nor] the policy of [the] administration"; he further thanked the bishop for his understanding cooperation and expressed the hope of counting him as an ally.[45]

The Catholic Daughters of America approached Gruening with a more specific petition: they asked that a Catholic consultant be named as head of the Social Services Department of Puerto Rico. Elitism and religious chauvinism were combined in their request. The Catholic Daughters stated that in Puerto Rico "the representative responsible and cultivated women are Catholics" and a Catholic would reject "meddling experiments" and respect the population's (that is, the elite's) disapproval of contraceptive practices. "Our women of good principles . . . do not consider Birth Control methods; the ignorant and irresponsible women accept Birth Control. Therefore Puerto Rico is spending money on unscrupulous and shiftless women which could be invested . . . in schools, orphanages, hospitals."[46]

Rumblings from the church, however, did not deter the Bournes. Even as these letters were being written, the PRERA was stepping up its birth control activities. In June 1935, Gladys Gaylord, executive secretary of the Maternal Health Association of Cleveland, Ohio, arrived in Puerto Rico at Dorothy Bourne's invitation. The purpose of the visit was to discuss further work in family planning. With Gaylord's help and that of Dr. José Belaval, a well-known gynecologist, and Dr. George Bachman, director of the School of Tropical Medicine, a trial birth control clinic began operating in July 1935.[47] Services were provided by Dr. Belaval, a second physician, and a social worker. The School of Tropical Medicine, an adjunct of Columbia University, provided the physical facilities, while the PRERA contributed the necessary personnel and contraceptive materials. At the end of six months the clinic had taken care of 104 patients, a work load that was considered "encouraging." In the words of Dr. Belaval, "The poor people had become so interested in the program that they flooded our clinic."[48]

The new visibility given to the PRERA's birth control activities stiffened both the opposition of the Catholic church and the federal officials' resolve to assuage or at least countervail the religious protests. Unlike the local lay organizations, which engaged in name calling and petty politicking, the church decided to treat the PRERA's stress on birth control as a symptom of Puerto Rico's ills and presented its own program for the island's economic rehabilitation. An extended report, "The Church and Reconstruction in Puerto Rico," was prepared by the Reverend R. A. McGowan, assistant director of the Social Action Department of the National Catholic Welfare Conference. The study on which the proposal was based was conducted in the summer and early fall of 1935 and had the approval of Monsignors Edwin V. Byrne, bishop of San Juan, and Aloysius J. Willinger, bishop of Ponce.[49]

In contrast to both the victim-blaming that characterized the Brookings study and the image of a carefree, shiftless population described by others, McGowan's report depicted a people conditioned by the helplessness of its colonial status and the pessimism of poverty. To those who discounted the capacity of the *jíbaro* for thrift and industry, the study pointed out that "thrift and industry cannot become habitual until persons have something to be thrifty with and industrious over."[50]

Addressing "the almost inevitable talk of overpopulation," the representatives of the church agreed with the Nationalists' position that this issue was being used to divert attention from Puerto Rico's more pressing problems. "It is a continuous recourse of the melancholy spirit. It excuses bad production, bad distribution, bad social organization and government inaction. It lulls to apathy. It excuses injustice."[51]

Instead of promoting "the deliberate under-production of human beings" to match the "deliberate under-production of physical things,"[52] the church sought to harness the island's economy "to make it serve its workers and the Puerto Rican people."[53] It therefore proposed a wide-ranging plan including

> greater production in Puerto Rico in products of the land and by preserving and processing them; . . . land distribution and higher wages as a condition of a better distribution of both the increased product and the present amount of production; credit, marketing and consumer cooperatives among the farmers to the same ends; labor unions to the same ends; a gradual but complete re-organization of the sugar industry to substitute forms of control which will make it serve the people generally; and the growth of local industries in whose ownership and control the cooperative element will be to the fore.[54]

Through this proposal the church clearly established that, unlike some of its lay leaders in Puerto Rico, it was not opposed to change, but rather favored a different economic system that would make population control unnecessary.

The conflicting political and economic ideologies espoused by the Catholic opponents of birth control were not lost on Edna Lonigan, one of the members of the technical committee that had studied the viability of the Chardón Plan. In a memorandum on birth control which combined demographic analysis with political acumen, she stated that "the Church is not a single unit, and that, back of the Church opposition in Puerto Rico, is the same old evidence of party politics using whatever emotional stresses there are to keep itself in power."[55] She also argued that changes in fertility did not depend only on the dispensing of birth control methods. "The chief element in a reduction in the birth rate is neither moral exhortation nor contraceptive devices. It is a mental shift, from a society in which the measure of satisfaction is survival, to one in which parents realize that they can raise the whole level of their children's lives by having fewer children and giving each of them more care."[56]

Nevertheless, Lonigan conceded that the economic rationale for birth control had little meaning in Puerto Rico. "To the Puerto Rican father ten children are ten sources of income. He knows that his neighbor with six children gets more wages from them than a man with three children."[57] She urged establishing a broadly based but cautious program of family planning based on eugenics and health promotion and carried out largely under private sponsorship. This involved three separate but closely related efforts:

1. Organization of a Race Betterment Association, to unite moderate Catholics and Protestants in a program to *improve racial stocks* in Puerto Rico, and to provide better care for children in their formative years, by emphasizing the *responsibility of fathers* in caring for their children, and raising the family's standard of living.

2. Extension of contraceptive information to individual mothers, through the maternity service of the Health Department, *only where such information is justified on medical grounds*.

3. Organization of a private Birth Control Committee to give technical contraceptive information and equipment, without *the slightest financial or administrative* connection with either Insular or Continental officials.[58]

Despite this advice and the fact that the PRERA had begun phasing out its activities in August 1935, Bourne continued the birth control program under the auspices of the FERA and the direction of Dr. Belaval, who proved to be an effective promoter of and lobbyist for birth control. At the 1935 annual meeting of the Puerto Rican Medical Association, Belaval was able to persuade his colleagues to approve a resolution requesting legislative action to permit the teaching and demonstration of contraceptive methods and the sterilization of the mentally deficient.[59]

Following a second visit by Gladys Gaylord in November of the same year, the PRERA instituted a large-scale island-wide birth control program encompassing services, research, and training.[60] Fifteen PRERA aides recruited women from all over the island. A candidate for the service would first obtain a health certificate from her local physician. Then a PRERA aide would take her to San Juan, where one of two types of contraceptive methods (foam or jelly) would be prescribed. Women who were unable to have their prescriptions filled in their hometowns would get the materials directly from the PRERA. Those who could not afford the materials worked for the PRERA to cover the bill.[61]

The research component involved experiments with the "natural period" (that is, the rhythm method), which had gained scientific respectability in 1933 following many years of contradictory and inconsistent evidence.[62] Training was carried out in San Juan as part of the activities of the original demonstration clinic. In December 1935 this clinic was moved from the School of Tropical Medicine to its own building, from which it provided services to the municipality of San Juan. Instruction on contraceptive methods was given to twenty-four doctors, fifty nurses, and seventy social aides. Within six months this new personnel was deployed in forty-five clinics operating in two-thirds of the administrative municipalities of the island. A total of 3,404 patients received birth control advice; careful records were kept for each of these and a strict follow-up system was instituted.[63]

Bourne and Belaval were planning to open a clinic in each of the island's seventy-seven towns, but on June 15, 1936, when they were most enthusiastic with their accomplishments, an order liquidating the FERA came from Washington. As a result, in Belaval's words, "the whole program of birth control came to a standstill; the personnel had to be discharged; and the clinics closed."[64] The contraceptive effort foundered in the bureaucratic shake-up, as it was later to collapse under political pressures.

The PRERA and the FERA for Puerto Rico were replaced by the Puerto Rico Reconstruction Administration (PRRA), which was directly accountable to Washington and worked with federal funds made available through the United States Treasury. The president named Dr. Gruening as administrator of the PRRA, and Gruening in turn appointed Dr. Carlos Chardón as the agency's regional administrator.

Although both Gruening and Chardón wanted to continue the program of birth control throughout the island, they were so busy organizing the new federal enterprise and initiating the scheme for agrarian reform that they were unable to give much attention to the "maternal health clinics." Toward the end of July 1936, however, the PRRA asked Dr. Belaval to reactivate the birth control project. With a budget of $250,000 for the first year, he was able to organize the work on a larger scale than before and planned to open sixty-one clinics.[65]

Aware of the need to mollify the church and preempt political opposition on this issue, Gruening decided to visit the bishop of San Juan, Monsignor Edwin Byrne, to discuss the proposed birth control program. Armed with facts and figures on the unemployment, poverty, and ill-health of the burgeoning Puerto Rican population, the PRRA administrator suggested creating a network of birth control clinics, "where good Puerto Rican Catholic mothers, who had had eight, nine and ten children but did not want to have eleven, twelve and thirteen, could get the necessary advice and information."[66] Gruening's presentation so persuaded the bishop that he agreed to "look the other way" if no publicity was given to the clinics.

Following this conspiratorial pact, the PRRA began opening maternal health clinics on the island. Fourteen clinics had been started when Gruening left for Washington "to report to the Congress on the progress of [the] reconstruction programs, confident that the birth-control clinics were an important part of [the] overall objective."[67]

A week later, the *Catholic Review* of Baltimore carried a front-page article written at the request of Bishop Byrne of San Juan. The article attacked the PRRA's maternal health clinics as "an insidious and sophisticated crime against God and humanity." While Gruening was wondering what had caused the bishop to break his word and reverse his stand, he received a telephone call from James Farley at the Democratic National Committee Headquarters. Farley was blunt and direct.

> "Gruening, what in hell is going on in Puerto Rico? . . . Whatever it is, stop it. We've had three bishops in here this morning. Have you seen this week's *Tablet*? (The organ of the Brooklyn Archdiocese.) Have you seen this week's issue of *America*? (The Jesuit Weekly.) Well, take a look at them. This is hurting us in the campaign. I'm going to Hyde Park tomorrow, and I want to be able to tell the boss that whatever we've been doing, we're not doing any more."[68]

With elections less than two months away, Roosevelt was naturally more intent on mending fences than on aiding economic reconstruction in Puerto Rico. Not one to jeopardize the president's reelection, Gruening was bound by both party discipline and policy directives to obey Farley's command. But first he had to confront Monsignor Byrne and find out why the bishop had stopped "looking the other way." According to Gruening, the bishop sighed and said, "I had no idea you'd do it on such a scale."[69]

Gruening later learned that was not the complete answer. Word of the PRRA clinics had reached Cardinal Hayes in New York, and he had called Bishop Byrne for an account of events in Puerto Rico. Cardinal Hayes was therefore able to exercise political power in Washington to impose Catholic morality in Puerto Rico. Moreover, he dealt a direct blow to his old adversary Gruening, who had attacked him in the *Nation* fifteen years before.

Following the conversation with Bishop Byrne, Gruening met with the social workers and medical staff of the PRRA and told them what had happened. He expressed his regret and said that no one on the administration's payroll could continue taking part in the birth control clinics.[70] Other staff members were informed that "legal technicalities" impeded the continuation of the program, and all work stopped on September 15, 1936.[71] Once again, Dr. Belaval was called upon to write an epitaph for this effort. "With no follow-up and no contraceptive material to be supplied to the patients, the 3,404 women treated were lost, and the work gone to the wind, as we could not reach any definite results regarding the cases."[72]

4. Private Initiatives and Legal Encounters

Those who had been most directly involved in the initiatives for the promotion of family planning on the island were unwilling to abandon the cause. This applied to the Puerto Rican promoters of these activities as much as to the outsiders. But their temporary setbacks also provided the occasion for the recruitment of new allies. News of the collapse of the PRRA birth control program traveled fast in the United States. Once Dr. Eric Matsner, medical director of the American Birth Control League, got word of it, he informed Dr. Clarence J. Gamble, who was on the league's board of directors.

Dr. Gamble, a physician by training, combined a researcher's intellectual curiosity with the gadgeteer's fascination with technology and the reformer's zeal for results. Moreover, as an heir to the Procter and Gamble fortune, he commanded plentiful resources with which to nurture his interests and support selected causes. In 1924 he became interested in contraception and decided to devote his professional life and philanthropic efforts to the cause of birth control.

Eager to promote this cause wherever it seemed necessary and the time ripe, Gamble saw Puerto Rico as an ideal place in which to test new methods and spread the practice of contraception. He was therefore quick to grasp the opportunity provided by the curtailment of the Puerto Rico clinics, and he wrote Gladys Gaylord and Dr. José Belaval to inquire about the possibility of developing a similar program under private auspices. He also dispatched his Smith College–trained "secretary of birth control," Phyllis Page, to Washington to talk with Dr. Gruening.

Gamble asked Gaylord if she would be able to go to Puerto Rico once again to help organize a birth control project, to which Gaylord replied that she did not think it necessary to send anyone down, since "there are outstanding Puerto Ricans in all fields who ought to be able to develop their own program.... They have enough training, knowledge of medical standards, to be able to direct the work and administer funds."[1]

Writing to Dr. Belaval, Gamble expressed his disappointment at the cancellation of the birth control program and his desire to maintain at least a demonstration clinic where statistics on the outcome of various contraceptive techniques could be collected. Gamble also indicated his willingness to cover part of the costs of operating such a center if this were planned and sponsored by "a committee of the leading citizens of San Juan."[2] Dr. Belaval, who was already planning to start a public clinic for the poor, gladly accepted Gamble's offer of financial support and his suggestion that "outside assistance" be sent to help organize the group.[3]

Gamble, however, did not wait for Belaval's response before sending Page to interview Dr. Gruening about the situation in Puerto Rico. Gruening was predictably sympathetic and told Page that "the government is pouring thousands of dollars into Puerto Rico and it's just as though they were pouring it into a sieve.... Birth control is the only hope."[4] He then explained how Catholic pressure had caused the preelection shutdown of the PRRA program and requested that his name not be mentioned in correspondence concerning birth control work in Puerto Rico. Asked how the Catholic opposition could best be met, Gruening said, "By going in as soon as possible and starting work—a boat leaves every Thursday and arrives Monday."[5]

In a meeting with Page in New York City, Dorothy Bourne communicated the same sense of urgency.[6] Exactly a week later, Page was on the boat to San Juan.[7] With Gamble's money, Gruening's tacit approval, and a list of names supplied by Bourne, she was indeed "going in and starting work." On November 22, 1936, a group of fifty interested persons met at the School of Tropical Medicine to plan the new birth control project. The constitution of the Asociación Pro Salud Maternal e Infantil de Puerto Rico (Maternal and Child Health Association) was presented, discussed, and adopted in substance. In addition, the group collected dues and elected officers. Estella Alcaide de Torres, founder of the second Porto Rico Birth Control League, was elected president; the other members of the board of directors included former governor James Beverley, Dr. José Belaval, several social workers (including some employees from the PRRA), and professors from the University of Puerto Rico. After the association had been duly constituted, Dr. Belaval announced Dr. Gamble's offer of financial support, which was accepted with a vote of thanks.[8]

In the early part of 1937 the Maternal and Child Health Association was able to open three clinics, each in a different environment and using a particular contraceptive method so that comparisons of the effectiveness of the various methods among the Puerto Rican population could be made. Two were in Protestant community hospitals, where Catholic opposition was a challenge rather than an obstacle.

Presbyterian Hospital provided facilities for a clinic in San Juan. Gamble sent two hundred dollars and a shipment of diaphragms so that this effort could get underway immediately.[9] The diaphragm seemed a promising method, and Gamble had been advised that its success in Puerto Rico would probably be higher than in the United States, "due to the lithe figures of the women, their long fingers, lack of inhibitions in regard to sex, and their teachability."[10] Those cases that could be adequately fitted were also provided with a contraceptive jelly (Lactikol B). At the San Juan clinic a physician did the initial pelvic examination and fitting, while a nurse followed up with periodic home visits.[11]

Another clinic was opened at Ryder Memorial Hospital in Humacao. This institution was sponsored by the American Missionary Association and the United Evangelical Church and staffed predominantly by United States physicians. The clinic prescribed Stoughton's foam powder and sponge and relied on patients' coming to the clinic instead of on outreach activities and house calls.[12]

After several months, Gamble became dissatisfied with the price of Stoughton's powder and turned to Johnson and Johnson as a possible source of supply. He proposed to test a new product in Puerto Rico and requested the pharmaceutical company's participation in a program that would provide it "the earliest information on the results obtained and the commercial value of knowledge that [its] material had been used ... in such a large-scale charitable enterprise."[13] Johnson and Johnson agreed to cooperate in the testing of a spermicidal powder in Puerto Rico and contributed fifteen hundred dollars to defray the expenses of the field trials.[14]

The third clinic, in rural Lares, was run by a nurse who had formerly been on the staff of Presbyterian Hospital in San Juan. This clinic prescribed jelly and syringe and made home visits to reach isolated patients. Some of these visits were made on horseback, although eventually the clinic obtained a mobile facility to broaden its clientele and scope of operations.[15] As a free-standing clinic with no back-up services, the Lares clinic instituted its own two-way referral system with the public health unit run by the Health Department, sending them patients with health problems and taking over patients recommended for "maternal health services."[16]

Uniform records and close statistical monitoring of the three pioneering clinics permitted an evaluation of the patients reached and the effectiveness of the contraceptive services provided. These resulted in a significant reduction in fertility: the preclinic pregnancy rate was 104 per 100 years of exposure to the risk of pregnancy, while the postclinic rate was only 40. Expressed in another way, the average interval between the end of one pregnancy and the beginning of another was lengthened from 11.5 months to 30 months using contraception. When those who had stopped using birth control were excluded, that interval stretched to 41 months. The differences in the effectiveness of the three methods studied were slight.[17]

In addition to these three pioneering clinics the Maternal and Child Health Association helped to get others involved in birth control activities. The association's prodding, coupled with postelection courage, reactivated the PRRA's efforts in maternal health. The agency provided aides for the association's clinics and supplied contraceptives and personnel for nine additional dispensaries.[18]

Another significant development was the opening of three birth control clinics on the plantations of the sugar companies. These were operated by the association though financed entirely by the *centrales*, each of which provided $150 per month for supplies and the services of a nurse.[19]

This alliance between the birth controllers and the sugar interests can be attributed to the convergence of several economic and ideological factors. The sugar companies were already introducing labor-saving technology that made the redundancy of workers increasingly obvious. Moreover, the message of the Brookings report had not been lost on them: population control was a way of reducing pressure on the island's limited land resources, thereby diverting attention from the increasing concentration of land into large holdings. It is also likely that the resident sugar entrepreneurs, as members of Puerto Rico's elite, shared the eugenists' view that excess breeding of the "inferior" stocks would inexorably lead to the deterioration of Puerto Rico's genetic endowment. Lastly, the owners of the sugar *centrales* must have realized that their survival depended on adaptive responses to social pressures, and birth control, however controversial, was more acceptable than redistributing the spoils of sugar through agrarian reform. Enlightened self-interest, rather than noblesse oblige or progressive attitudes, can therefore account for the support of family planning by this particular group.

With the help of the Protestant community hospitals, the PRRA, and the sugar estates, the Maternal and Child Health Association had a set of flattering statistics to report upon completion of its first year of service to the cause of birth control: it had opened fifteen clinics and taken care of 2217 patients.[20] Gamble felt he had obtained an adequate return on his investment; although the total patient load was small compared to the needs of Puerto Rico, he reported, it represented a more rapid rate of growth than that of any other clinic group.[21]

The delivery of contraceptive services, however, constituted only part of the association's activities. The group was equally involved in changing the legal and social climate under which services were provided. This required lobbying for the repeal of the Comstock Laws and the enactment of legislation that would further the dissemination of contraceptive knowledge and practices.

In 1937 the association effectively catalyzed the introduction of three key pieces of legislation which had been drafted by the Health Department.[22] Law 116 provided for the creation of the Eugenics Board to consider compulsory sterilization for medical or moral reasons. Law 133 amended the penal code to eliminate the clause that made the dissemination of contraceptive information and practices a felony. This legislation, which had been advocated by Dr. Lanauze and the Ponce Birth Control League in 1925, had been introduced and defeated periodically during the intervening period. Law 136 authorized the commissioner of health to provide maternal health and birth control services through the island's public health centers.

Although the three pieces were viewed as a package, Laws 133 and 136 elicited the most controversy and opposition. In addition to having the strong support of the Maternal and Child Health Association, these bills had the public backing of the commissioner of health, the Puerto Rico Medical Association, and the Graduate Nurses' Association, as well as that of many social workers, university professors, and civic leaders. Through testimony and quiet lobbying these groups were able to secure the support of the speaker of the House, the president of the Senate, and the only woman member of the legislature.[23] Together, they were able to override the bitter opposition of the Catholic church and lay organizations, and the legislation was approved by both houses in April 1937.

The critics of the bills saw this as only a temporary setback. Their next tactic was a pressure campaign aimed at Governor Blanton Winship, who possessed veto power over the legislation. Brandishing the specter of rampant immorality and invoking the "red scare," Bishop Byrne requested that the governor veto the bill. "If our Government now legalizes immorality, may God help and have pity on us all. Then our government will be following the lead of Communist Russia which also has legalized Birth Control. For the moral prestige of our United States, for the moral prestige of Christian Puerto Rico, please save us from such a national shame."[24] The bishop also encouraged the distribution of petitions in favor of a gubernatorial veto, which were signed by thousands of parishioners.

The ever-militant National Catholic Welfare Conference sent a copy of Monsignor Byrne's letter to President Roosevelt, urging him to intervene to insure that Winship would not approve the legislation.[25] The Puerto Rico chapter of the Catholic Daughters of America similarly addressed the president, informing him that the bills that had been approved had been "made by unscrupulous men for unscrupulous men" and denouncing the proposed legislation as an invitation to promiscuity. "Birth control measures in the hands of . . . ignorant people would only make them a prey to disease and to men of loose morals confident of no evil consequences to themselves. We who know the characteristics of our people and we who deeply wish Puerto Rico to be a country of high standards, deep principles and good morals are afraid of our future."[26]

To counteract the pressure from the Catholics, the Maternal and Child Health Association launched its own campaign in favor of the ratification of the bills. Estella Torres asked Clarence Gamble to cable the governor and to get other birth control leaders to do the same.[27] Gamble urged Governor Winship to approve the bill "for physicians' freedom and vital service to mothers and children" and wrote Margaret Sanger requesting that she send a similar message.[28] James Bourne also wrote a letter of support.[29]

This barrage of letters, cables, and requests left the governor in a quandary. While he favored the proposed legislation, he was particularly sensitive to the Catholics' accusation that a Protestant governor had no right to impose his ideas on a Catholic country.[30] Winship consulted Ernest Gruening, who devised a stratagem to secure passage of the bills while saving the governor's face. Dr. Gruening's advice was simple but clever: "Leave Puerto Rico and appoint Rafael Menéndez Ramos, the Commissioner of Agriculture, as acting governor. . . . He's a devout Catholic, but he'll sign the bill. Then it will have been the work of a Catholic House, a Catholic Senate and a Catholic Puerto Rican governor."[31] Governor Winship followed Gruening's counsel, and when the controversial bills reached the governor's desk on May 1, 1937, it was Menéndez Ramos who signed them into law.

In a cautious statement justifying his support for the bills, the acting governor indicated the need to subordinate religious misgivings to the economic, medical, and humanitarian arguments for birth control. Concerning the first, Menéndez Ramos stressed the grievous limitation of federal aid in the face of "undesirable and unbridled procreation, especially among the poor and less cultured strata of [the] population." Scientific and humanitarian birth control would attack the problem at its source, reducing the unemployed multitudes who lacked an opportunity to earn decent livings.

The medical reasons favoring birth control were basically eugenic, aimed at doing away with the "inferior stock" that had haunted true believers in race betterment.

> In Puerto Rico, as well as in all countries of the world, there is a considerable portion of the population which, because they are victims of certain incurable and hereditary diseases, should abstain from bearing offspring who, born with the unavoidable stigma of an unfortunate heritance, would be condemned to endure a miserable and unhappy life. In a more or less distant future, these unfortunates would fill our reformatories, sanitariums, and insane asylums. These children can not, in any way, contribute to the happiness of their parents and much less to the general economic and social welfare of our people.[32]

The third rationale for contraception concerned the welfare of mothers, for whom "the noble mission of motherhood [was] a sad and inevitable martyrdom." This statement did not have a feminist thrust, however; rather, it was an extension of the economic argument, rooted in the need to regulate the birthrate among poor peasants.

Menéndez Ramos concluded his explanation by underlining the fact that it was not an appointed governor from the United States who had signed the birth control bill into law. "We understand that the consensus of the Puerto Rican Legislature conveys the sentiment of the majority of our people. It is, therefore, of a significant, historical coincidence that the responsibility of signing this law should have fallen upon a Puerto Rican."[33]

The enactment of the birth control bills gave legitimacy to the activities of the Maternal and Child Health Association at the same time that it made them virtually unnecessary. The Health Department could now absorb the existing program into its regular services and provide contraceptive information and methods throughout its network of public health units.

This plan was forestalled, however, by one final counterattack by the Catholic opposition. The Catholics argued that Law 136 violated a federal obscenity law prohibiting the use of contraceptives in any United States territory. Since the legislature of Puerto Rico was empowered to pass only those laws not contrary to acts of Congress, they maintained that the federal law supervened.[34] Once again, the uncertainties and ambiguities of Puerto Rico's relationship with the United States inhibited the island's freedom of action.

Dr. Eduardo Garrido Morales, the commissioner of health, intended to begin an island-wide birth control program on July 1, 1938, and the sum of twenty-five thousand dollars had been allocated for this purpose in the budget for fiscal year 1938–39.[35] Nevertheless, Dr. Garrido was loath to proceed without an opinion from the office of the U.S. attorney general confirming the legality of the Puerto Rican statutes. "In the event that such an opinion cannot be obtained," he wrote Dr. Gruening, "I wish you would make an effort to have a bill introduced in Congress, providing for an amendment to the Federal statutes that would eliminate any question as to the Insular legislation on this subject being in conflict with the Federal legislation."[36]

Dr. Garrido also sought the advice of two physicians from the U.S. Public Health Service. They felt that it would be unwise for the Health Department to promote an intensive contraceptive program for two reasons. First, it would have no great effect upon the total population, for any decrease in the number of births, they said, would simply improve the chances of more babies surviving to maturity.[37] Furthermore, the doctors had little faith in the efficacy of the existing methods and in the sophistication of those agreeing to practice them. "There is no absolute method of preventing conception (except continence) so that under the best possible conditions, with birth control widely advocated and practiced by the doctors of the Insular Department of Health, and accepted by ignorant and uneducated women, the birth rate would not be profoundly affected."[38]

Second, it would antagonize a powerful religious group. The physicians argued that the clergy could be of great help to the Health Department in public health education and that this beneficial relationship should not be jeopardized by one phase of the department's varied program.[39]

To clarify the ambiguous legal situation, the doctors suggested that perhaps it would be worthwhile "for some local physicians ... to arrange to be arrested for giving contraceptive information and let the Courts determine whether or not any United States law is being violated."[40]

By June 1938 the board of directors of the Maternal and Child Health Association knew they were heading toward a legal showdown. Although they had continued to open new clinics and were operating a total of twenty-two, the Catholic opposition had grown. The district attorney for Puerto Rico, Cecil Snyder, informed Estella Torres that he was getting daily letters and appeals asking him to enforce the old federal law prohibiting obscenities and contraceptive materials in the territories. Another federal law prohibited cockfights, a popular Puerto Rican amusement, and it was felt that public support for birth control might be secured by maintaining it in the same questionably legal category as cockfighting.[41]

Faced with the health commissioner's reluctance to provide birth control services without a clear legal mandate and the sugar manufacturers' unwillingness to continue sponsoring activities tainted by illegality, the leaders of the Maternal and Child Health Association felt that, in the absence of a favorable opinion from the U.S. attorney general, they had no option but to provoke a test case.[42] District Attorney Snyder consulted Attorney General Homer S. Cummings, who ruled that the federal statute applied and ordered the district attorney to institute proceedings against the Maternal and Child Health Association. Snyder, who was personally friendly toward the birth control movement, met with the board of directors of the association to work out a strategy for clarifying the legal situation. Carmen Alvarado, the association's executive secretary, wrote Dr. Gamble about the outcome of the meeting.

> It has been decided that a raid in our clinics is not the best thing ... because it will attract publicity and will probably deprive us of the valuable help of the PRRA, private hospitals, municipalities and centrals cooperating with us. We will submit evidence in a few good cases so as to avoid the raid. The members of the [Board of Directors] will be prosecuted for sponsoring the movement and also a doctor ... for doing the actual work.
>
> The trial will take place before the judge alone. We want to avoid the jury in order to avoid publicity. As individuals, we don't fear publicity in this respect, but ... the agencies cooperating with us do fear it and we want to save our clinics above all.[43]

Dr. Gamble, who was very much interested in obtaining a favorable decision in this case, secured the legal counsel of Morris Ernst, a prominent New York attorney. A defender in civil liberty and obscenity cases, Ernst had won a significant victory in 1936 in a case concerning the importation of pessaries.[44] Ernst assigned a colleague to the Puerto Rico case and submitted a detailed brief to Dr. Gruening. The attorneys argued that the proceedings in Puerto Rico were unnecessary.

> If the problem were one for which there was no legal precedent, the government might well take the position that it was constrained to institute proceedings to clarify the legal situation. However, this is not the case. The question of the legality of the dissemination of birth control information and the giving of contraceptive advice in proper cases has been favorably passed upon by the courts, directly and indirectly, in numerous instances.[45]

Citing six cases supporting "the proposition that birth control advice may be legally given by licensed physicians where proper medical indications exist," the lawyers urged that the authorities in Puerto Rico be instructed accordingly.[46]

The New York counsel advised their Puerto Rican clients to limit their defense to the medical aspects of the cases, and not to mention population or economic questions at all. Accordingly, the association chose to be judged on the services rendered to four high-risk, high-parity mothers for whom additional pregnancies would mean probable death.[47]

The case went before a grand jury in December 1938. Writing to Dr. Gamble two weeks before, Torres was hopeful for a no true bill and a minimum of publicity. "I am hoping that the Jury will not find cause for inditement [sic] as the cases Dr. Belaval has selected are splendid ones, and Snyder will base his case on these four examples. If they do indite [sic], he has promised to keep the case as quiet as possible and avoid all unnecessary publicity."[48] Dr. Gamble was less sanguine about the outcome of the case. He discussed the possibility of birth control work being "entirely impossible" in the aftermath of the trial, but sent his best wishes to the members of the association and the hope that "I shall not have to visit you in jail."[49]

On December 16, 1938, the federal grand jury returned indictments against six directors of the Maternal and Child Health Association. In addition to doctors José Belaval and José Caso, those indicted were Estella Torres, Elsie Domenech (married to Governor Winship's economic adviser), Ana Laura Delgado, and Celia Núñez de Bunker (director of social work in the Department of Education). The newspapers underlined the social prominence of the persons involved and the legal importance of the test case.[50]

By arrangement between counsel, it was decided that a stipulation of facts would be presented to U.S. District Judge Robert A. Cooper for a trial without a jury. The defense submitted its brief in written form, and the federal case took scarcely ten minutes.⁵¹ Judge Cooper rendered his opinion on January 19, 1939. While deciding that the federal statute was applicable to Puerto Rico, he nonetheless upheld the validity of Laws 116, 133, and 136 except for one section of the latter which permitted contraception for social and economic reasons. Citing legal precedent in the United States—particularly the case concerning the importation of pessaries—Judge Cooper argued that "it can hardly be successfully contended . . . that a physician is prohibited from giving contraceptive advice and materials in a case where, in good faith and in the exercise of reasonable skill, he believes it is necessary for the preservation of life or health."⁵²

Section 5 of Law 136, which explicitly allowed the provision of contraceptive information to persons whose poverty or poor living conditions did not permit the adequate rearing of children, was found to be in conflict with the prevailing federal statute and was therefore struck down. Thus the judge concluded that

> while I think it is not only the right but the duty of a physician, when in his judgment such is necessary for the protection of life or health, to prescribe contraceptives, nevertheless, anyone, whether physician or layman, who gives advice or furnishes drugs or other devices for the sole purpose of preventing conception, will be subject to prosecution and punishment.⁵³

In summary, the ruling sustained the applicability of federal legislation in Puerto Rico, affirmed the right to disseminate contraceptive information for health reasons, upheld the overall validity of Laws 116, 133, and 136, and found the defendants not guilty.

Although Judge Cooper's opinion restricted the scope of the activities of the Maternal and Child Health Association, no such restriction occurred in practice: many of the women seeking birth control advice were suffering from tuberculosis, anemia, and other diseases, and the prescription of contraceptives was in fact regarded as "necessary medicine."⁵⁴ Moreover, there was a high correlation between illness and poverty, and the social and economic indications for contraception were indirectly taken into account by the providers of birth control services, who tended to interpret the law in a liberal manner.⁵⁵

The decision was therefore hailed by the Maternal and Child Health

Association, who could look back on a creditable record of service and two noteworthy legal triumphs. Between early 1937 and June 1939, the association had advised more than five thousand women in twenty-three clinics and undertaken several research projects.[56] More important, it had finally made it possible for the Department of Health to embark on a large-scale birth control program.

5. Uphill!

Scarcely a fortnight after Judge Cooper's decision, Dr. Garrido Morales began "making preparations to start birth control work in [the Health Department's] different hospitals, antituberculosis centers, public health units and rural dispensaries."[1] The legislature appropriated funds for the purchase of materials and equipment for this work, and the commissioner of health attempted to intimidate the bishop of San Juan by telling him that his opposition to birth control would make him "the most hated man in Puerto Rico for generations to come."[2]

Still, administrative and financial obstacles restricted the extension of family planning services throughout the Health Department. Although there were no less than 139 facilities where birth control clinics could be organized, the effort required guidance from the central level.[3] The work was placed under the direction of the department's Bureau of Maternal and Infant Hygiene, which had ample authority but limited personnel.

Much of the bureau's effort was focused on supervising and regulating the services provided by *comadronas*, or midwives, who handled 80 percent of all births.[4] Since 1931 the practice of midwifery had been restricted to those who were licensed by the Health Department. Women who identified themselves on birth certificates as assisting in deliveries were legally required to submit to training organized by the department or face prosecution for the illegal practice of midwifery. After training and licensing the *comadronas*, who were usually illiterate women, the Health Department attempted to supervise their activities through monthly case conferences and continuing education programs that stressed the importance of asepsis and taught the rudiments of obstetrics.[5] The *comadronas* practiced on a fee-for-service basis, receiving money or payments in kind directly from their patients. For obvious reasons, this cadre of health workers could hardly be expected to promote birth control. Instruction on contraception was therefore assigned to the few nurses who worked under the direct supervision of the head of the Bureau of Maternal and Infant Hygiene.

Financial constraints also limited the availability of services. By 1939 the flow of reconstruction funds had dried up and Puerto Rico had not been included in the health programs enacted under the Social Security Act. Secretary of the Interior Ickes described the attitude of the U.S. Congress toward Puerto Rico as one of "lack of interest and even actual hostility";[6] as a result, the island failed to benefit both from regular federal programs and from special congressional appropriations. Belaval had to inform Gruening that the birth control work would be reduced to one-fourth its present level if outside help was not forthcoming.[7]

"Outside help" indeed arrived, although through an unexpected and circuitous route. In 1939, Governor Winship played host to two U.S. senators from the South. While staying at La Fortaleza, the governor's palace, their wives took ill with diarrhea, and Dr. Garrido Morales set up a makeshift hospital in the governor's mansion. While ministering to the wives, Garrido told the senators that Puerto Rico was in dire need of additional resources for the provision of health services. Upon their return to Washington, the senators were able to secure Puerto Rico's inclusion under titles 5 and 6 of the Social Security Act, which provided federal grants-in-aid to the states for maternal and child health and for crippled children's health services. This decision, which became effective in January 1940, increased the budget of the Health Department by fully one-third and allowed for the extension and intensification of practically all health activities.

Birth control activities were one of the principal beneficiaries of the influx of federal funds, enabling the public sector to take over major responsibility for this service. Although the Maternal and Child Health Association retained clinics in San Juan, Humacao, and Yabucoa, its executive secretary and a number of specially trained nurses joined the Health Department. Dr. Belaval became the medical director of the expanded governmental program, which provided contraceptive advice in all public health units and rural subunits of the island.[8] By June 1940 the Health Department had recruited additional public health nurses and social workers, and had opened sixty prenatal and infant hygiene clinics in nineteen municipalities.[9]

Garrido's windfall had no counterparts in other spheres of Puerto Rico's economy, and the initial impact of the New Deal weakened, as programs were phased out and projects were discontinued. Moreover, some of Roosevelt's progressive legislation proved counterproductive when applied to Puerto Rico. The Fair Labor Standards Act, passed in

1938, sought to help workers by abolishing child labor, setting wages above the starvation level, and regulating working hours. The act created the Wage and Hours Division within the Department of Labor to oversee the enforcement of adequate minimum wages. The administrator of this division had full power to investigate any manufacturer and to enforce standards through the courts.[10]

In Puerto Rico the effect of the wage-and-hours bill was disastrous: instead of protecting labor, it killed most of the industries and increased unemployment.[11] The needlework industry was particularly affected. The quintessence of "women's work," this industry operated on a piecework basis, employing thousands of women who worked at home and delivered embroidered handkerchiefs and linens to entrepreneurial middlemen. For the rural female population the wages earned through this labor—however meager—represented a means of subsistence during the *tiempo muerto*. Unable to operate competitively at the mandated wage rates, this industry declined significantly, leaving thousands without jobs.[12]

As the 1930s ended, Puerto Rico's economic picture was as bleak as it had been a decade earlier. Only the rate of population growth showed a sustained and uninterrupted rise throughout the period.[13] Despite the depressed economic conditions, the death rate had declined, while the birthrate remained fairly stable at around 39 per 1000 inhabitants. The population rose 2 percent per year, while economic opportunities stagnated or shrank. Although the labor force increased at a rate of 10,000 per year during the thirties, agricultural employment declined: in 1940 the number of jobs in this sector was lower than it had been in 1930 and even less than it had been in 1910.[14]

The situation had become so critical that several high-powered lobbies, including the Chamber of Commerce and the Farmers' Association, requested that President Roosevelt name an interdepartmental agency to survey conditions in Puerto Rico. The president complied in May 1939 by appointing a committee composed of representatives of the departments of State, Interior, Agriculture, Commerce, and Labor and the Tariff Commission.

The staff report to the Interdepartmental Commission on Puerto Rico, dated September 9, 1940, urged the immediate adoption of a policy on population control. Indeed, the concern with excessive numbers was a leitmotif throughout the report:

> Steps should be taken [to reduce] the birth rate . . . at least to the level of the death rate. . . .[15]
>
> A balance between needs and means cannot be struck without a drastic change in present population trends; . . . without widespread and determined resort to birth control.
>
> Unless the population problem is solved, all else is whistling in the wind. In that sense it is literally true that the population problem is THE problem of Puerto Rico. Birth control is by no means the only remedy for the Puerto Rican problem, but it is that remedy without which all other remedies are mere palliatives and will prove futile as a permanent solution.[16]

This report was never adopted by the presidential group, however, so it remained as yet another descriptive document concerning Puerto Rico's plight.

The problems of landlessness, land monopoly, and absentee ownership persisted, demonstrating that federal funds, policy commissions, and technical committees were no substitute for leadership and direct action. Whatever "solutions" had been tried had been costly and ineffectual. The decade of the forties thus ushered in a number of interrelated changes. These included changes in political leadership as well as institutional changes, both of which were conditioned and constrained by the climate brought about by war.

In the political sphere the changes revolved around the person of Luis Muñoz Marín. Muñoz, who alternated between being a keen observer and political commentator and an active participant, realized that the previous failures could be utilized to wrest political power from the existing leadership. In 1936 he had broken with the leader of the Liberal party, Antonio Barceló, over electoral strategy and the quest for independence.[17] When U.S. Senator Millard Tydings proposed a bill offering Puerto Rico a plebiscite on the question of independence, Barceló opted for the bill and for independence. Muñoz, however, found the bill unacceptable: it would condemn Puerto Rico to independent famine, an unreasonable price for political freedom. The issue was submitted to an intraparty vote, and Barceló won.

Muñoz refused to reconcile himself to his defeat. He began organizing the conservative independence wing of the Liberals into a group called the Acción Social Independentista and attempted to capture the party machinery. By May 1937 the differences between the two groups had sharpened and continued coexistence became more and more unlikely. At a party convention held that month the majority of the Liberals approved a resolution expelling splinter groups from the party. Muñoz was left with a small group of supporters and no political apparatus through which to channel his ambitions. But nature and nurture had made him a politician, and he had advanced too far to settle for an ignominious retreat. He therefore decided to launch his own party.

On July 22, 1938, the Popular Democratic Party (PDP) announced its registration in two voting districts, thereby gaining recognition as a new and distinct political entity. Its symbol was the profile of a *jíbaro* wearing the traditional straw hat; its battlecry, "Uphill!" Its slogan was "Bread, land and liberty." The placement of these three words was not fortuitous, but rather reflected Muñoz's conviction that political freedom was a meaningless abstraction for the people of Puerto Rico until they had conquered hunger and gained control over their land. The problem of Puerto Rico's political status was thus subordinated to the island's more immediate economic problem.

Between 1938 and 1940 the PDP launched an intensive campaign based on clean elections and a policy of "fair shares" for the dispossessed poor, particularly those in the rural areas. In the absence of a party organ and access to the news media, Muñoz and his followers relied on their own canvassing efforts. Appointing local leaders throughout the island, Muñoz combed the countryside for potential constituents. Addressing them in small groups, he stressed two fundamental points: that the island's status must not be an electoral issue, because status could not solve the problems of the people, and that the people must not sell their votes, for by doing so they abdicated their right to participate in their government.[18]

Accordingly, the 1940 PDP platform downplayed the status issue and highlighted the measures required for economic development. Agrarian reform was the most important element in the proposed program. A key plank was enforcement of the five-hundred-acre law, along with redistribution of agricultural land and government regulation of the sugar mills.[19] The program also included a variety of "New Deal"–style reforms: the enactment of a social security system of unemployment, disability, old age, maternity, and sickness insurance; slum clearance; and the establishment of an official system of low-interest loans for workers and the middle class, among others.[20]

On election day the PDP received approximately 215,000 votes, about 38 percent of the total. The new party won ten of the nineteen Senate seats and eighteen of the thirty-nine House seats. With a majority of one in the upper chamber, the PDP proceeded to name Muñoz, who was elected senator-at-large, president of the Senate. He thus occupied the principal position of political leadership in Puerto Rico.[21]

Despite this victory, a coalition of the Republican and Socialist parties won a plurality of the votes cast in 1940. In the legislature, this alliance won control of the same number of House seats as the PDP and one less Senate seat. It thus lost the legislative control it had enjoyed for eight years, but remained a strong opposition party, one which Muñoz's *populares* could not easily dismiss. A third political party, the Tripartite Union, won three House seats; it therefore held the balance of power in the lower chamber and could decide whether or not the PDP legislation would be approved.[22]

Muñoz Marín's power effectively depended on exercising party discipline in the Senate and convincing one of the minority representatives to join the PDP stalwarts in the House. In addition, he relied on the sympathies of the governor, who had veto power over bills and a direct line to Washington. Fortunately for Muñoz, Governor Blanton Winship had been replaced at La Fortaleza in 1939 by Admiral William H. Leahy, who was in turn succeeded by Guy J. Swope. Neither of the latter two remained in office long enough to constitute a menace to the Senate leader.

Muñoz's political ascent undoubtedly restricted the choice of a new governor in Puerto Rico. Following Muñoz's victory, Secretary of the Interior Ickes sent Rexford Tugwell to Puerto Rico as the head of a study team investigating methods of enforcing the five-hundred-acre law.[23] Coupled with his previous experience and his stated willingness to be "on call" if Roosevelt had real need for his services, this assignment made Tugwell an appropriate candidate for the vacant governorship.[24] He was designated for the job in the spring of 1941 and sworn in on September 19, 1941.

In many ways, Tugwell was significantly different from his predecessors. He was familiar with Puerto Rico and had exercised administrative leadership in Washington and New York.[25] He recognized the need for bold action. Because he believed that "the world [was] a laboratory" and trial and error an acceptable method of experimentation, he regarded Puerto Rico as promising terrain for new ideas of development and management.[26] The fact that in Puerto Rico everything remained to be done was a spur to creativity. Surely, the "stricken land" he had visited in 1934 and 1941 had little to lose from his experiments. Furthermore, Tugwell entered a political milieu different from that which his predecessors had encountered. Muñoz's role as Senate president assured that.

Although both the popular press and certain historians have characterized Tugwell and Muñoz Marín as a team and emphasized their similar outlooks and complementary skills, the contrasts between the two leaders were as striking as they were deep. Usually described as dark and brooding, Muñoz's appearance reflected his literary past rather than the political present. Wrinkled suits and large-plaid shirts were his sartorial trademarks. Tugwell was known for his well-groomed appearance and immaculate attire, both of which were targets of political commentaries and press caricatures.[27] The men were equally dissimilar in personality. Even though both were articulate and urbane, they presented varying images to the public. Tugwell was, according to one biographer, "warm and engaging in private, ... blunt and outspoken in public."[28] Muñoz was ruthless and impatient with his associates but infinitely charming with the electorate, addressing crowds in language that *Time* magazine said was designed to "go straight to the heart and mind of the humblest and least educated hearer."[29]

Ideologically, both men were oriented towards the use of government intervention to control economic forces for the achievement of desired ends.[30] They were also committed to Puerto Rico's development; their personal reputations, as much as the island's welfare, were at stake. Nevertheless, the planner and the politician operated within different time frames and had different constituencies. These considerations led to differing priorities, strategies, and tactics. In the words of *Time* magazine, "Tugwell could never get over the fact that Muñoz acted sometimes like a high-minded idealist, sometimes like a job-hungry political boss. Muñoz, on the other hand, found it difficult to convince Tugwell that even an idealistic politician needs enough patronage to grease the machine and win the next election."[31]

Yet both men were pledged to the same program and shared the same enemies. They realized that noncooperative efforts on their part would only keep Puerto Rico mired in the petty politicking and sense of helplessness that had characterized the island's political and economic life for decades. In addition, Puerto Rico was facing the crisis of World War II, which gave a sense of urgency to all governmental activities and cut the island off from its main source of imports. Besides their perennial problems, Puerto Ricans had to deal with food and fuel shortages, rampant inflation, and labor unrest. Charles Goodsell summarized the situation as follows:

> From November 1941 to November 1942 prices jumped 53 percent compared to 16 percent on the mainland. Inflation, in turn, caused serious strikes, beginning in January 1942. As public works projects were cut back, and as industries laid off workers because of a lack of

imported raw materials and shipping space to export produced goods, unemployment shot up—from 99,100 in July 1941 to 237,000 in September 1942.[32]

Puerto Rico commanded a critical position in the military defense of the Western hemisphere. As the buildup of German U-boat activity disrupted shipping in the North Atlantic and threatened the security of the Panama Canal, the island became an important staging ground for United States naval and air force operations. Nevertheless, Tugwell was determined to keep the war from becoming an excuse "to take people's minds off injustice and to prevent any change which would threaten their privileges."[33] In his first message to the legislature, he therefore announced his resolve to push on with the social changes that were long overdue. Developed in consultation with Muñoz Marín, Tugwell's program was designed to create the machinery of government needed for reform.

The legislation proposed in 1942 sought to rival the scope and pace of Roosevelt's first one hundred days, which established the legal underpinnings of the New Deal. In Puerto Rico, Tugwell's foresight and Muñoz's ability to convince and bargain secured the enactment of a total of forty-three bills. In a single week no less than seven major public institutions were created.[34] Two of these—the Planning Board and the Puerto Rico Development Company—were tributes to Tugwell's belief, expressed in his message to the legislature, that Puerto Rico's limitations existed "far more in men's minds and in their organization than in any rule imposed by nature."[35]

The Planning Act as drafted by Tugwell and his associates provided for a board with island-wide jurisdiction over land use and public expenditures, both to be regulated in accordance with a master plan. Projected improvements would be locked "into a logical whole which could be broken with difficulty."[36] The act reflected Tugwell's conception of planning as a "fourth power," incorporating elements of the executive, legislative, and judicial functions but possessing an independent power of its own.[37]

Thus the proposed law contained provisions to protect the agency from executive and legislative interference. Both the agency's scope and its independence were curtailed before the law was enacted, however. All rural areas were exempted from zoning and other land-use controls, and the board's projected autonomy was emasculated by requiring the legislature to approve all plans and regulations. Despite these modifications, Tugwell considered the law to be "a fairly modern one" and "extremely useful."[38]

The creation of the Development Company (Fomento) was based on the governor's opinion that development was not going to occur through private enterprise without increased public direction or encouragement. Government intervention was required to "gather up Puerto Rican capital and help to direct its uses, together with the energy of the people, into channels which will yield livings for all.... New industries can be brought by government to the pilot-plant stage and then shared, sometimes, with private or semi-public capital; or perhaps cooperatives can be encouraged."[39] The statutory powers and responsibilities of Fomento were consequently varied and far-reaching: they included carrying out research on the marketing, distribution, and manufacture of potential products; making loans to industrial and commercial enterprises; promoting private investment; and establishing public manufacturing enterprises.[40]

The political and institutional changes catalyzed by Muñoz and Tugwell had ramifications affecting practically all aspects of Puerto Rican life. Whereas previously no one had looked to government for the solution to problems, government now emerged with the power to initiate, prod, and build. This marked the beginning of paternalism—and the creation of a new type of dependency.

The new regime had implications for population policy and birth control. In his inaugural address, which stressed the need to alleviate conditions at home even while preparing for a struggle abroad, Tugwell specifically rejected population control as a means to reduce poverty. Instead, he favored the tapping of underutilized resources to meet the menace of "that favorite frightener, overpopulation."[41] At the same time, he placed himself in the eugenists' camp by supporting selective breeding.

> Certainly it cannot truly be said that the Island is overpopulated so long as its resources have not been fully utilized and brought to the people.... The responsibility put upon us by the fertility of the people must be met with plans for greater production.
>
> This does not imply that society should forego its interest in encouraging increase among the healthiest of its citizens and discouraging increase among the obviously unfit. But it does suggest that the easy alibi of overpopulation which excuses neglect, lethargy, and selfishness is not one into which we should allow retreat without challenge.[42]

Even allowing for the rhetorical flourishes and hortatory nature of inaugurals, this statement evidently represented a departure from Tugwell's previous advocacy of population control. Tugwell's subsequent writings provide several explanations for the apparent about-face. First, unlike those who advanced birth control as a way of preventing the bearers of bad stock from multiplying and diluting the gene pool, Tugwell felt that a policy of contraception would probably by dysgenic, leaving "the worst human stock [untouched] while the better stock reduces its contribution to the future population."[43] Moreover, he was an optimist concerning the possibilities of increasing the goods available to meet the needs of growing numbers. He thus rejected the existence of a fixed "quantitative ratio between the food supply and the numbers there are to use it."[44] In Puerto Rico, nature's very profligacy buttressed his conviction that "there must be a way of fixing everything else."[45]

In addition, Tugwell regarded overbreeding as a symptom of a people in despair, "like a sick tree which flowers desperately out of season in the attempt to perpetuate its race when its own individual survival seems unlikely."[46] Economic improvement would make people provident by giving them a greater stake in their future and a vested interest in their children's well-being. Birth control was thus a by-product rather than a prerequisite of development. Lastly, by 1941, Tugwell's understanding of the intricacies and dynamics of social systems had made him skeptical of attempts to control complex processes through the manipulation of a single factor. Both his training and experience led him to see the significance of parts only in relation to the whole; population policy therefore had to be subordinated to the broader goals of increasing productivity and redistributing wealth.[47]

The commissioner of health whom Tugwell appointed to replace Dr. Garrido Morales, Dr. Antonio Fernós Isern, shared the governor's views on the population question. Fernós favored birth control as a eugenic and public health measure, but felt that the promotion of contraception would have a negligible effect on population growth. Such factors as the organizational difficulties of reaching the rural population, the ignorance of the potential beneficiaries, and the casualness with which many Puerto Ricans entered into marital relationships, particularly consensual unions, hampered the success of a family planning program. Fernós strongly condemned the practice of concubinage and recommended raising the legal age of sexual consent among women. Blaming Puerto Rico's economic system for the apparent surplus of inhabitants, he characterized the prevailing plantation economy as one which "degrades the human personality . . . by transforming workers into slaves."[48] He therefore held that the population problem was really a problem of stunted development and urged "the economic and political decolonization of the island, without which Puerto Rico's economic and industrial development is impossible."[49]

Given this ideological position, the new commissioner of health had little interest in dispensing birth control services. Furthermore, because of a long-smoldering quarrel with Garrido Morales, Fernós was reluctant to support a program that had been so clearly identified with his predecessor. Initially, Fernós opted to change the form more than the content of the program. In a clear demonstration of the demise of the "old order," he ordered the destruction of educational brochures on birth control and the elimination from the program of some contraceptive devices.[50] When Belaval submitted a series of recommendations to improve the services, Fernós's only action was to insert a new preface into the handbook of instruction on contraception.[51] The program was subsequently reorganized and allowed to languish.

> The specially trained and enthusiastic nurses inherited from the Asociación were relieved, and the work was assigned to the general public health nurses in addition to their other numerous duties. Physicians as a rule were not interested in birth control and tended to leave it entirely in the hands of their assistants. Personnel shortages resulted in a severe curtailment of all follow-up activities.[52]

While official health policy did little to boost birth control, general development policy sought to encourage family limitation. The Planning Board's guidance and intelligence systems called for the close monitoring of demographic trends. Changes in the size, composition, and distribution of the population were therefore documented and analyzed. The agency's second technical report focused on Puerto Rico's "population problem"; it recommended that the Health Department increase its family planning case load by ten thousand to twenty thousand cases per year in order to reach a total population of three hundred thousand. The estimated cost of $7.50 per case was considered to be a minimal price to pay for the stabilization of the Puerto Rican population for a period long enough to allow more fundamental factors—for example, higher standards of living and universal education—to act on the birthrate.[53]

Fomento was similarly concerned with the rise in population. The "take charge" mystique that it tried to promote concerned both production and reproduction. The agency's chief aim was to create jobs, and it feared that the gains made in industrial employment would be wiped out by increases in the labor force. Statistics on new employment opportunities were useful for public relations purposes, but the leadership recognized that the acid test of Fomento's effectiveness was its impact on the unemployment rate. It thus had a legitimate interest in keeping the denominator down.

The conflicting policies espoused by the governor and the Commissioner of Health, on the one hand, and the planning and development apparatus, on the other, were further complicated by the impact of World War II. The war had far-reaching and contradictory effects on the politics and practices of population control. Moreover, it transformed the societal environment within which decisions concerning reproduction were made.

In 1940, Eleanor Roosevelt had lent her prestige to the birth control movement by publicly declaring her approval of family planning. The following year she invited leaders of the movement and representatives of the Public Health Service, the Children's Bureau, and the Department of Agriculture to discuss "the general outlines of the proper governmental approach to public health and population problems."[54] In October 1941 the Surgeon General's Office announced that the Public Health Service would consider a state health department's request for funds for a "child-spacing program," and in 1942 the surgeon general indicated his approval of planned parenthood programs.[55]

This change in federal policy—which affected the services financed by Title 5 funds in Puerto Rico—cannot be attributed solely to pressure from the White House. When the United States entered the war, the health and productivity of the female population became very important. Since many vital industries required women workers and unwanted pregnancies removed workers from the assembly lines, the provision of birth control services became part of the war effort. As a result, in May 1942 the Public Health Service began actively to promote contraceptive programs.[56]

Ironically, the same war conditions that transformed birth control into a social necessity and even a patriotic duty made contraceptives increasingly difficult to obtain. The Puerto Rico Health Department's annual report for fiscal year 1942–43 indicated that some 142 clinics had been operating and 6,242 cases had been seen. Yet the report also stated that war conditions had limited the availability of contraceptive materials, and produced a decline in the number of new admissions.[57]

More significant, the war increased the frequency and intensity of cultural interchanges between Puerto Rico and the United States. Prior to the war, exposure to the mainland culture had been limited for most of the Puerto Rican population. During the war the two peoples had numerous opportunities for exchange. Thousands of American servicemen were based in Puerto Rico; an even larger number of Puerto Ricans went to the mainland to serve in the armed forces. The expansion of defense installations on the island meant that Americans and Puerto Ricans worked side by side. In addition, the war had a profound impact on two socioeconomic phenomena—industrialization and migration—that laid the basis for Puerto Rico's postwar development effort.

6. The "Battle of Production"

The law that created Fomento in 1942 gave that agency a broad mandate to start and promote new activities through a variety of mechanisms. These included setting up a wholly owned corporation, selling part of the stock of subsidiaries to the public, issuing bonds, and entering into joint efforts with private entities. Because the new agency inherited a successful cement factory begun under the auspices of the Puerto Rico Reconstruction Administration, Tugwell could report that Fomento was "a going concern from its day of organization."[1]

In addition to the versatility of its legal authority and the inheritance of the PRRA, Fomento had the advantages of dynamic leadership and adequate finances. Teodoro Moscoso, a pharmacist by training, was selected to launch Puerto Rico's industrialization program. Moscoso had managed his family's drugstores before entering government service. In 1938 he was appointed director of the Ponce municipal housing authority; Tugwell, noting his performance, promoted him out of Ponce and into the governor's office as coordinator of insular affairs.[2] His abilities thus successfully tested, he was the governor's choice to direct Fomento.

An increase in rum revenues gave the organization the finances it required for takeoff. When the production of distilled liquor was curtailed in the United States during World War II, the demand for rum for export soared and rum factories in Puerto Rico increased their production. At the same time taxes on all spirits were raised. Since revenue taxes on goods shipped from Puerto Rico to the United States reverted to the insular treasury, for several years Puerto Rico had a return of revenues that almost doubled the island's income. Tugwell succeeded in sequestering these funds, which were later used to finance Puerto Rico's development efforts.[3]

Originally allocated five hundred thousand dollars and the cement plant, Fomento shortly received an appropriation of $20 million. This money enabled the company to build and operate several factories and within five years there were five plants in operation: the original cement plant, a glass bottle factory, a carton plant, a shoe factory, and a clay products factory. Funds were also committed for a $7 million resort hotel and a $4 million textile mill.[4]

As the war ended and the rum bonanza tapered off, Fomento's program came up for appraisal and readjustment. The cement plant had produced a handsome profit, but this was not enough to offset the losses sustained by the remaining Fomento subsidiaries. These had been plagued by shortages and delays in the acquisition of machinery and materials, lack of managerial and technical know-how, marketing problems, and strikes.[5] In addition to being financial failures, the government enterprises had failed to make a dent in the island's unemployment problem. By the end of fiscal year 1947, $20 million had been spent and only 845 jobs had been created by the five Fomento plants.[6] This total represented less than 1 percent of the new employment opportunities that were needed on the island.[7]

In the face of dwindling finances and a disappointing record in the creation of jobs, Fomento shifted its course from state capitalism to the promotion of private industry in manufacturing. The Aid to Industrial Development Program, established in 1945, assisted private investors in starting new projects by providing part of the required investment. This assistance consisted primarily of the construction of factory buildings for sale or lease to private manufacturers. Thus Fomento acquired the land and provided the physical plant for industries, while private firms furnished equipment, working capital, and managerial expertise. As the gradual change from government-owned enterprise to the promotion of private investment became official policy, government officials argued that the new course would broaden the effectiveness of the capital at Fomento's command, secure experienced management, and take advantage of the existing marketing channels of established organizations.[8]

As Fomento began to promote Puerto Rico to U.S. businessmen, the five original subsidiaries became an embarrassment. Not only were they unsuccessful but they also smacked of socialism.[9] The relative importance of these pioneering efforts was muffled as Fomento used the pages of *Fortune* and other magazines to extol the advantages of locating industry in Puerto Rico. In Moscoso's words, as early as 1945 the leadership of Fomento had realized that "the resources of the insular government in themselves would not be sufficient to solve the problems that lay ahead" and therefore had sought help from outside.[10] The new strategy represented a commitment to the use of U.S. capital, and hence to the continuation of Puerto Rico's ties to the United States. What Puerto Rico had to offer was an unlimited supply of cheap labor.

The political implications of Puerto Rico's development strategy were discussed by Muñoz Marín in a series of articles published in the newspaper *El Mundo* in February 1946. In the first of these he defined the problem facing Puerto Rico as that of an increasing gap between population and resources. Prior to 1934, he wrote, Puerto Rico's productivity had kept pace with its population growth. After that date, however, production had leveled off, while the population had kept increasing at an accelerated rate, reaching fifty-five thousand per year by 1945. While this situation would normally have resulted in a decline in the per capita share of the island's economic product, this had not happened in Puerto Rico: an increase in federal aid had cushioned the effects of the economic decline, meeting the demands of the additional thousands of mouths to feed, children to educate, and families to house.[11]

Puerto Rico also had to cope with the effects of a demographic transition. In the long run, Muñoz argued, rising incomes and improved living conditions would result in lower fertility and smaller families. In the short run, however, these improvements only lowered the death rate while leaving the birthrate untouched. This of course resulted in a rising rate of natural growth and in an increase in the number of inhabitants beyond the capacity of the island's economic resources. Muñoz estimated the number of persons that were being "artificially supported" by federal aid and other temporary economic measures at five hundred thousand.

In 1922, Muñoz the journalist had advocated contraception as the means to attack the "monster of overpopulation." Now, however, Muñoz the politician favored an increase in production as the solution to the population-resources problem. "What we have to do ... is: increase production, within the standards of justice, with the speed required so that our increasing population may reach full employment, and higher standards of living, without the artificial help which has sustained its life since we exceeded the figure of 1,600,000 inhabitants."[12]

In a second article, entitled "The Program," Muñoz defined the eclectic, experimental nature of the development program on which the Popular party had embarked. The program had to rely on both public initiative and private enterprise, eschewing the ideological constraints imposed by the choice of one over the other. Similarly, expertise and help were welcome regardless of their source, whether from within or outside Puerto Rico.[13]

In a final essay, "Political Status," Muñoz underlined the need to solve Puerto Rico's political problem without jeopardizing its economic survival.[14] Differentiating the island's position vis-à-vis the United States from colonial relationships in which the wealth of the colonies was used to enrich and improve the standard of living in the dominant nation, Muñoz stated that the United States had acquired Puerto Rico by mistake rather than out of greed. Given this historical perspective, he concluded that political freedom would not automatically result in the island's economic betterment. Rather, an independent Puerto Rico would not be able to sell its products in the world's largest and most prosperous market, thereby stifling the island's potential for industrialization.[15] The tension between political freedom and economic protection was thus explicitly recognized, though left unresolved.

Since 1943, Muñoz had given much thought to a compromise status that would provide some type of self-government yet guarantee economic assistance. After the New Deal, the volume of federal funds reaching Puerto Rico was roughly equal to the yield from the largest crop.[16] Independence therefore meant the loss of a major source of income. For Muñoz, this situation constituted an ideological conflict and a personal dilemma; in Tugwell's words, "Muñoz was fairly caught between his old *independentista* sentiment and a new conviction that Puerto Rico could not exist except with United States support."[17]

The end of World War II and the advent of the atomic age gave Muñoz a new outlook on the status question. The global scale of political conflict and the menace posed by the new weaponry, he contended, required a rethinking of basic political concepts; "sovereignty" and "freedom" had lost their meaning in a shrinking world in which, increasingly, interdependent nation-states were required to bargain away their absolute authority in exchange for freedom from fear.

In June 1946, Muñoz was ready to propose a new political formula aimed at bringing about the elusive goal of "self-government without the slavery of the threat of hunger."[18] In his quest for "new roads toward old objectives," he rejected both independence and statehood. Instead he proposed three formulas for consideration: self-government under the prevailing conditions until the economic situation permitted a plebiscite on independence and statehood; an immediate plebiscite conditioned on granting the chosen status when a given economic standard was achieved; or full autonomy, with the proviso that the Puerto Rican legislature could conduct a plebiscite on status when it so chose.[19] While indicating no particular preference, Muñoz urged the quick adoption of a concrete solution to the problem of the island's political identity and expressed the hope that all parties would support the proposed change in status.

That change would take another six years, however; in the meantime, Muñoz and the PDP devoted themselves to Puerto Rico's development efforts. In July 1946, Muñoz once again addressed the population question. At a round-table discussion held by the Puerto Rico Public Health Association on the topic "Puerto Rico's Population Problem," government officials, academicians, and public figures presented their views on the subject. When the proceedings of this meeting were published, Muñoz Marín was invited to write an introduction. In it, Muñoz stated that the population problem was perhaps the most serious problem facing Puerto Rico, but was cautious concerning possible solutions.

> Our aim must be to increase our production more rapidly than our population. . . . To achieve this, several solutions are offered. I am not in favor of all that are proposed. Besides, probably none would be sufficient by itself because the problem is grave and urgent. It seems to me that the principal solution lies in . . . the "battle of production," which the government has already begun in industry and agriculture.[20]

As Fomento struggled to attract industry and Muñoz made the "battle of production" the core of the PDP's program, many Puerto Ricans were waging the battle elsewhere: in Manhattan's garment district, in the streets of the South Bronx, and the steel mills of Lorain, Ohio. During World War II, the War Manpower Commission made arrangements for the recruitment of more than two thousand Puerto Rican laborers to work in occupations connected with the war effort. The availability of jobs in the United States, combined with the lack of opportunities on the island, said Commissioner of Labor Manuel A. Pérez, resulted in many workers eagerly enrolling "in any migration movement, regardless of its destination or the terms of the proposal."[21]

Following the war, thousands of Puerto Ricans chose to emigrate. Approximately sixty-five thousand Puerto Ricans had served in the U.S. Armed Forces; many of these were stationed in the United States, Europe, Africa, and Asia. Some decided to stay in the United States once the war was over; others returned to the island only to migrate to the United States with members of their families.

If the war was instrumental in breaking down the psychological barrier to emigration, transportation technology was even more important in accelerating and facilitating the outward movement of population. Whereas the first groups had relied on passage on the S.S. *Marine Tiger*, the inauguration of direct air service between New York and San Juan in 1946 transformed the situation of the potential migrant. The process of uprooting and transplanting individuals and even families became deceptively simple and inexpensive: travel time was reduced to seven hours; travel costs fell as low as ten dollars for a one-way ticket between San Juan and New York.[22] The results of this were immediate: in 1945, 13,500 Puerto Ricans entered the city; in 1946, almost 40,000. As a result, according to Nathan Glazer and Daniel Moynihan, "New York was in the middle of a mass migration rivaling the great population movements of the first two decades of the century."[23]

While this exodus was unprecedented in its scale and intensity, it did not represent an entirely new phenomenon in Puerto Rico. As early as 1900–1901, there had been eleven expeditions of Puerto Ricans to Hawaii. A total of 5,000 persons emigrated at the expense of Hawaiian planters, who spent $565,000 for passage and recruiting costs.[24] The experiment was hardly a success. As Harry Hirschberg was to observe, "The lightly clad Puerto Ricans suffered from the cold in San Francisco and some died enroute; many were taken to hospitals in Hawaii and some died there."[25] Culture shock and restlessness on the part of the immigrants and unmet expectations on the part of the planters led to a number of clashes, and the number of Puerto Ricans employed on the plantations fell from 3,206 in 1902 to 1,907 in 1905. The report of the commissioner of labor of Hawaii for the year 1905 concluded that, as a result of this experience, "the experiment of importing Porto Ricans . . . is not likely to be repeated; and those who are at present in Hawaii will doubtless continue to constitute a decreasing fraction of the plantation force."[26] A second group, however, left Puerto Rico for Hawaii in 1921, and the 1930 census indicated a total of 6,671 Puerto Ricans in Hawaii.

In 1926 two groups of Puerto Rican emigrants went to work in the cotton fields of Salt River Valley, near Phoenix, Arizona. As had been in the case of Hawaii, adjustment problems led to their return or eventual dispersal, and the hope that such a movement would "relieve a very serious condition in Porto Rico and also answer a purpose [in Arizona]" did not materialize. Thus the general manager of the Arizona Cotton Growers Association wrote to General McIntyre, chief of the Bureau of Insular Affairs, on August 30, 1928: "The condition of the Porto Ricans that are still in Arizona . . . is not what I would call satisfactory. . . . They do not fit into our Arizona life in a way that would encourage more to come; what they think of Arizona undoubtedly is not favorable, and what Arizona thinks of them as a whole is likewise."[27]

These disappointing experiences, however, did not discourage emigration altogether. By 1940 there were close to seventy thousand persons of

Puerto Rican birth living in the continental United States, most of these in New York City.[28] Another sizable group had settled in St. Croix, where the similarities of climate, occupational structure, and life-style eased the transition and led to a successful adjustment.[29]

After 1945 emigration appeared increasingly feasible to the individual and desirable to the body politic. Fomento's efforts at job creation had neither kept pace with the increases in the labor force nor accommodated the underemployed workers in the agricultural sector and those displaced by the greater mechanization of cane production. Even the advocates of Muñoz's "battle of production" maintained that Puerto Rico had an excess population of half a million; the hope that the promise of industrialization would be fulfilled still seemed illusory. As the exodus of Puerto Ricans increased from a trickle to a steady stream and later to a flood, public officials began to think of emigration as a "safety valve" to relieve the island's economy of part of its labor surplus. While tact and pride prevented the Puerto Rican government from overtly encouraging emigration, its development strategy required a population outflow. In the words of Glazer and Moynihan, "The island government needed emigration as well as economic development to cope with [its] problems; if it did not encourage emigration directly (an unnecessary provision), it planned for and assisted it."[30] This planning and assistance took three forms: influencing the composition of the emigrant group, diversifying the possible destinations, and providing services to the migrants during the settlement process.

Attempts to affect the composition of the population leaving the island took place after a study conducted in 1947 showed that emigration constituted a "brain drain" and had an adverse effect on the skills of the population left behind. Clarence Senior's study of the Puerto Rican emigrants found that the population movement was selective of the better educated. The emigrants included more skilled workers than the average for the island, and the average education of those leaving was higher than the average for those remaining in Puerto Rico. The survey also found that the main purpose of the trip was to seek employment and that males predominated among those leaving.[31]

The government of Puerto Rico therefore tried to promote the emigration of low-skilled women. According to a report prepared for the Caribbean Commission this would not only balance the distorted sex ratio but also "relieve the present unemployment situation . . . and assure [a] long-term beneficial effect by helping to reduce the birth rate."[32] To accomplish this, a training course was offered for Puerto Rican women wanting to enter domestic service in the United States. The first course, which was begun in October 1947 on an experimental basis, included sixty women "carefully selected to meet certain recommended qualifications for work in the States."[33] This effort, however, was on too small a scale to have much of an impact.

Although the exportation of population represented a "brain drain" for Puerto Rico, many of the emigrants were socially and economically disadvantaged in the United States. Besides their language difficulties, they often had less schooling and fewer skills and were able to find employment only in the lowest rungs of the occupational ladder. They were also darker and poorer, and thus forced to live in the blighted slums of New York and other cities. Not surprisingly, they formed ghettos and were stigmatized. Tugwell's racist comment in 1933 was proving to be prophetic: the incoming Puerto Ricans indeed made up a "wave of the lowly," and they were, in U.S. terms, "poor material for social organization."

Concerned with the unhappy lot of the emigrants and aware of the discrimination to which many were subjected, Puerto Rican officials gave serious consideration to the possibility of diverting them to other countries in the Caribbean and in Central and South America. Because of its proximity, the Dominican Republic seemed a likely destination and one that was repeatedly studied with care.

After the Chardón Plan emphasized the need to reduce Puerto Rico's population and advocated the promotion of large-scale colonization projects, the president of the Dominican Republic, Rafael Leonidas Trujillo, made President Roosevelt a tentative offer in 1936.

> If you believe that it is not practicable to obtain the land necessary for the execution of your plans in Puerto Rico, ... and if, at the same time, you believe that the Puerto Rican problem could be properly solved by diverting part of its excess population to the Dominican Republic, where the state has extensive and fertile tracts of land of its own for the settlement of families of farmers, which would be offered to them on extremely advantageous conditions, I do not doubt that the obvious thing would be to formulate a plan which, while providing the solution of a problem which is vital for Puerto Rico, would give rise to close relations between two peoples whose destinies are identical as to tradition, race, and language.[34]

On the basis of this offer, United States secretary of state Cordell Hull instructed the U.S. Dominican legation to submit a memorandum on the subject.³⁵ The letter accompanying the report warned that Trujillo's motives could be suspect, for he knew "that considerable sums of money [had] been appropriated by the American Government for the rehabilitation of Puerto Rico and hope[d] that part of these funds [could] be utilized for the benefit of [the Dominican] Republic as well as Puerto Rico."³⁶ In addition, the proposed scheme had a number of serious drawbacks, including the fact that the political conditions in Santo Domingo were unsatisfactory compared to conditions in Puerto Rico and that it appeared that the Dominican Republic would welcome in substantial numbers only Puerto Ricans who would pursue agricultural activities and whom that government would regard as "white."³⁷ Hull therefore urged caution and further investigation before committing the U.S. government to any plan that would facilitate the migration of Puerto Ricans to the Dominican Republic.³⁸

Trujillo's proposal, scuttled in 1936, was revived in 1945 when a Dominican official approached Tugwell with the suggestion that Santo Domingo accept a large number of Puerto Rican immigrants in exchange for favored markets in Puerto Rico.³⁹ Tugwell sent Raymond Crist, a professor of economic geography at the University of Puerto Rico, to do a survey of the uninhabited and thinly settled areas of the Dominican Republic where Puerto Ricans might be resettled.⁴⁰ In the middle of his survey, however, Dr. Crist was recalled at the request of the State Department, which was worried about its relations with Trujillo at that time.⁴¹ Nevertheless, the geographer had studied the situation enough to conclude that a mass colonization scheme in Santo Domingo was not practical under the existing regime and that those who would best adapt to the new conditions would be the least likely to leave Puerto Rico. "There is a real opportunity in the Republica Dominicana for those who have a little capital, and who wish to settle on small owner-operator farms. This is, however, the type of person who is already successful in Puerto Rico, and who would be little likely to think of emigration."⁴²

Despite these objections, members of the U.S. Congress and even the Office of Puerto Rico in Washington continued to advance similar proposals. These contemplated, in addition to the emigration of Puerto Ricans, a commercial treaty giving trade preference to Santo Domingo and the development of a U.S.-subsidized agricultural resettlement project on Dominican soil.⁴³ Although these proposals received due consideration from a number of people—including President Truman⁴⁴ and top officials from the departments of State, Interior, and Agriculture⁴⁵— they were eventually turned down on logistical, economic, and political grounds. A Brookings Institution survey of the capacity of the Dominican Republic to absorb immigrants placed the feasible number at five thousand—far less than the hoped-for figure of sixty thousand or even six hundred thousand proposed by some advocates of the resettlement scheme.[46] Furthermore, any trade concessions granted by the United States to Santo Domingo would violate the most-favored-nation treaties entered into with other countries and would be contrary to the U.S. policy of lowering trade barriers and doing away with trade preferences.[47] Finally, the proposals posed important political problems: they involved loss of U.S. citizenship to the emigrants and assumed a continuation of Puerto Rico's political status. It was also feared that other Latin American republics would "cast aspersions at an expedient which might be construed as U.S. inability to deal positively with the problems of its dependent territories."[48]

As the opportunities to develop an "overseas province" in Santo Domingo receded, officials in San Juan and Washington probed other countries, including Venezuela and Costa Rica, on their willingness to accept Puerto Rican colonists. These countries usually mentioned finance, politics, and race as the main impediments to any proposed large-scale immigration.[49]

Undaunted by the rejection of their overtures, Puerto Rican officials formed the Emigration Advisory Committee chaired by the secretary of labor and composed of top-level political figures and public servants, including Luis Muñoz Marín, Teodoro Moscoso, and Clarence Senior. This group was in close contact with Dr. Fernós Isern, who had left the Department of Health to become resident commissioner, Puerto Rico's representative before the U.S. Congress.

In his new position, Fernós was spending a considerable amount of time and energy in Washington dealing with the problems arising from Puerto Rican emigration to the United States.[50] In August 1947 he had written the *New York Times* to comment on the island's exportation of population. Using medical metaphors to characterize the problem and its solution, he described Puerto Rico as suffering from "hypertension" and requiring a "good emergency 'bloodletting' scientifically carried out." Otherwise, a "spontaneous hemorrhage"—the current population movement—would occur. He went on to stress the national scope of the problem and the possibility of planned intervention in the migratory process.

Neither Puerto Rico nor New York City should be called upon to take care of this matter by themselves.... It should be the nation's concern. On the other hand, emigration may not be forced on free citizens; it may only be stimulated and regulated. If the proper conditions are found to exist in any given place and the proper inducements are offered, emigration will of itself start and develop. It could be done in such a way as temporarily to relieve Puerto Rico of the results of the present acute disproportion between its population and its available resources.[51]

As Puerto Rico's man in Washington and self-appointed apologist for the emigrants in the United States, Fernós was particularly desirous of finding alternative destinations for the population outflow. He was therefore not reluctant to employ measures best classified as "heroic medicine." When the State Department began planning for the colonization in the Western Hemisphere of four hundred thousand displaced persons still living in camps in Europe, Fernós suggested "mixing in" Puerto Rican emigrants among the Europeans to be resettled.[52]

This suggestion was discussed by the members of the Emigration Advisory Committee, who finally agreed that, "while the matters [of resettling the displaced persons and the Puerto Ricans] might well be presented jointly to Congress and other Washington authorities, ... it would be highly undesirable to try to mix the two groups in the actual colonization efforts, and ... it probably would be more satisfactory to place them in separate colonies."[53]

No proposal, however absurd, was dismissed outright. Other possibilities examined by the committee included establishing a Puerto Rican colony in the valley of the San Francisco River of Brazil, resettling families on banana plantations in Surinam, and exporting labor to work in the oil refineries of Curaçao.[54]

Some of these schemes received more thorough attention. Moscoso, whose Fomento was not hamstrung by cumbersome rules and regulations concerning what it could and could not do, dispatched a representative to Brazil to examine the viability of establishing a colony in the interior of the country. He reported that the environment was too hostile and the salaries too low to prove attractive to the Puerto Rican population.[55] In addition, Brazil had a "white only" policy with regard to immigrants.[56] A final hurdle was the cost of resettlement, estimated at around five thousand to six thousand dollars per family.[57]

Foiled in this attempt to decrease Puerto Rico's redundant labor force, Fomento opted for a more modest plan: it subsidized the national airline of Costa Rica (LACSA) in an attempt to lure Puerto Ricans to relocate to Central America. This, however, proved to be ineffectual.[58]

These futile gestures dimmed the hope of deflecting the migratory stream away from the United States. Instead, the Office of Migration was created to monitor job opportunities in the States and to distribute the emigrants in places other than New York City. Operating under the aegis of the Puerto Rico Department of Labor, the office also offered orientation programs, job-placement services, and training. While disavowing the overt promotion of emigration, this agency eased the process of acculturation by serving as middleman between Puerto Rican workers and prospective employers and providing a variety of supportive services to the arriving immigrants.

In 1948, when the office started operating, it had a large and growing clientele. That year approximately 260,000 Puerto Ricans were already in the United States, and the northward flow was continuing.[59] There was no doubt that Puerto Rico was exporting a significant part of its population; what could be disputed was the desirability of this measure. The *popular* leadership, who believed in winning the "battle of production" at home even at the expense of those abroad, feared that the transfer of population was at best a temporary expedient. As *Time* reported, "Island officials have a recurrent nightmare in which the U.S. undergoes a business recession and the Puerto Ricans, who as unskilled workers would be the first to be fired, swarm back to their homeland."[60]

7. The TVA of the Tropics

These nightmares and others no less traumatic rapidly began to disturb the sleep of Puerto Rico's political leaders and that of the vigorous new administrators who were recruited to manage the "battle of production." As indicated earlier, many of the Puerto Rican emigrants were severely handicapped in their new setting. The language barrier and their lack of marketable skills limited their opportunities; the jobs they were able to secure within the American labor force therefore tended to be not only the least desirable but also the most susceptible to the fluctuations of the economy. When thrown out of work with the onset of recession, many would abandon the urban slums and the rigors of the winter cold to return to Puerto Rico. As a result there were pronounced cyclical ups and downs in the net rate of out-migration.[1] Migratory statistics on Puerto Rico became as sensitive an indicator of the fluctuations of the American economy as boxcar loadings, capital goods inventories, and other such measures used by Wall Street analysts.

Despite the uncertainty of external events, a comprehensive strategy for remaking Puerto Rico into a modern society evolved. Piece by piece, Puerto Rico's new leaders were able to create the institutional mechanisms that assured the development of the island as a competitive industrial workplace fully integrated into the American market system. In less than a generation a traditional agrarian society was converted into one which was technically oriented, highly industrialized, and, essentially, urbanized.

This transformation was remarkable for its rapidity, the depth of its penetration, and the diversity of the areas affected. Major political and economic changes converged with profound alterations in the social, cultural, and demographic conditions of the island's population. Change in one area fueled change in the others, thereby enlarging the scope of the process and accelerating its pace.

The offensive that the government mounted was designated "Operation Bootstrap." As the agency involved in attracting industry to the island,

Fomento became the most visible arm of that campaign. The Fomento managers were both promoters and "institution builders." Through a combination of tax incentives, the recruitment and training of a labor force, the construction, sale, and rental of factories, and the creation of the financial and technological services that industry required, they were able to create an environment of assured profitability for mainland venture capital. This required sustained commitment and an ever-broadening public relations effort. Because Puerto Rico's major asset was its exploitable labor force, the island attracted chiefly the stabilized or declining industries that had to rely on cheap labor to survive.[2]

Many of these succumbed to reduced markets and increasing wages, and Fomento had to constantly renew its efforts to create new jobs and replace those that were being lost. In its campaign to attract industry Fomento converted one of Puerto Rico's apparent disadvantages, that of location, into a developmental asset. In a number of instances, the island's location between sources of raw materials and the market for its products was successfully promoted to corporate interests. The program was responsible for the creation of 120,000 jobs, representing more than one-seventh of the current labor force.[3]

The organized effort to encourage postwar development also tapped other sectors of Puerto Rico's economy. The island's climate, scenic beauty, and cultural diversity were the basis for a major expansion of tourism. In its promotion of Puerto Rico as a tourist haven, the government employed the same kind of incentives and an even more lavish display of the public relations skills that it had used to encourage industry. Tourist dollars became an increasingly important source of income. The assistance that the government gave to the development of tourism was not, however, unrelated to its concern for the promotion of industry, for it involved creating an environment which would be familiar and attractive to American businessmen and technicians taking up residence on the island.[4]

The government also tried to encourage the diversification of agriculture both to reduce dependence on food imports and to develop the production of additional farm commodities for overseas trade. It directed particular effort to the improvement of livestock production, the cultivation of pineapples for canning, and the creation of a modern poultry industry. Results, however, were disappointing.[5] In fact, Puerto Rico's long-standing dependence on imported food supplies continued to increase. In recent years more than four-fifths of all foodstuffs consumed on the island have been supplied from overseas, primarily the United States.[6]

Even while the leadership assembled and put into operation the separate programmatic elements that fueled Puerto Rico's rapid economic upsurge, a profound demographic change was occurring. An extensive public health and medical-care system had been slowly built up during the first four decades of American rule. Although the health status of the population had been significantly improved, Puerto Rico remained a disease-ridden island that still lacked many of the essential sanitary controls most often taken for granted elsewhere. Malnutrition, associated with the widespread poverty of the thirties, aggravated the severity of the many infectious diseases that ravaged the population. In 1940 the crude death rate stood at 18.4 per 1000 and the average life expectancy at birth for both males and females was only forty-six years. Especially appalling was the infant mortality rate, which exceeded 113 deaths during the first year of life for every 1000 live births.[7]

The two decades from 1940 to 1960 were witness to a remarkable improvement in the health status of the population as measured by traditional indices of mortality. The death rate dropped to 6.7, lower than that for the United States, life expectancy increased to almost seventy, and mortality among infants was more than halved.[8] Never before in human history had a society experienced such a rapid rise in its survival rate.

Life was made safer and more certain primarily through the control that was secured over infectious disease. Malaria was eradicated, tuberculosis was contained, and other infectious diseases were attacked through an expansion of the government's measures to sanitize the environment and provide personal health services. In 1940 diarrhea and enteritis, tuberculosis, pneumonia, and malaria collectively accounted for more than half of all deaths. By 1960 less than one-fifth of a much smaller total could be attributed to these four disease categories.[9]

This recital of statistics not only testifies to a basic alteration in living conditions but also bespeaks a fundamental change in the prevailing orientation of the population. In less than a generation, it became possible for persons to accept life itself with a new sense of confidence. As life became less of a precarious domain dominated by unfathomable hazards, persons found powerful incentives to adopt a more future-oriented outlook, eschewing the island's prevailing fatalism and the concern with otherworldly beliefs.

The improvement in the island's health convincingly demonstrated the efficacy of scientifically prescribed practices. Such a rapid change in the way life is experienced inevitably promoted alterations in expectations as well. Persons not only became aware of new possibilities but were sensitized to the kind of rational calculation necessary to take advantage of them. One of the first attitudes to change was that concerning family size, as persons began to recognize the greater likelihood of children surviving to adulthood. The control achieved over mortality also made the population more receptive to the idea of family planning.

But a far more apparent result, at least to those who viewed unchecked population growth as a societal problem, was the major surge the decline in the death rate precipitated in the rate of the natural increase of the population. During this period the birthrate remained as high as it had been in previous decades, for some years peaking even higher. Like many other countries, Puerto Rico experienced a postwar "baby boom." Family formation which was interrupted or deferred during the war years surged, as though making up for lost time. Accordingly, the marriage rate rose and the birthrate increased to the unprecedented levels of 42.3 in 1945, 42.6 in 1946, and 43.2 in 1947.[10] Even when the number of births leveled off, the enormous reduction in the level of mortality greatly increased the rate of natural increase.[11] The excess of the birthrate over the death rate, which was already large, increased by approximately half its former amount.

This substantial spurt in the biological rate of population increase was of course masked by the massive emigration of Puerto Ricans to the United States. Because of this out-migration the island's population grew slightly slower during the decade of the forties than it had during the previous ten years. During the next decade migration reduced the growth of the island's population even more effectively. From 1950 through 1959 net emigration is estimated to be have totaled between 430,000 and 470,000 persons.[12] Since Puerto Rico's population at that time was not much in excess of 2,000,000, during that decade every fifth Puerto Rican abandoned the island in favor of the United States.

Migration thus served to spare Puerto Rico the full demographic consequences of the drastic reduction in the death rate between 1950 and 1960. In the absence of migration the population of Puerto Rico would have approached an annual rate of increase of 2 percent during that period; because of the massive outflow of the fifties, the rate averaged less than 0.6 percent per year during that decade.[13] Table 7.1 summarizes the demographic circumstances underlying the island's continued economic growth.

These demographic changes were important for the economic changes brought about by Operation Bootstrap. The government's program of industrial promotion would not have succeeded without the improvement in the health status of the population that came after 1940. Persons debilitated by malaria and other infectious or parasitic diseases cannot be made into productive factory workers. Conversely, they could not have been so rapidly freed from their heavy burden of disease except for the changes in their living conditions that came with postwar industrial and urban growth. Rising incomes, improved nutrition, protected water supplies, dramatic increases in literacy combined to create not only a new certainty about life itself but new ways of living and new hopes. The control that was won over disease was a complex achievement, both product and producer of the chain reaction of innovation that engulfed the society.

Emigration also altered the scope and character of the development process. Besides reducing the rate of population growth, it withdrew large segments of the reproductive population, hollowing out the groups fifteen to forty-four years of age. This exodus contributed to a rising per capita income and prevented extremely high rates of unemployment on the island.[14]

The creation of a healthier population, together with the extensive postwar movement between the island and the United States, was accompanied by far-reaching social and cultural changes that further contributed to Puerto Rico's transformation. Three of these warrant special attention because of their potential role in family planning: the increasing participation of women in the labor force, the adoption of middle-class values, and the growing cultural exchange between Puerto Rico and the United States.

As Fomento sought to capitalize upon the cheap and willing labor in a grossly underemployed population, it took advantage of a hidden asset.

TABLE 7.1. Total Population of Puerto Rico and Selected Demographic Indicators, 1930–1960

	Total Population[a]	Rate per 1,000 *during the Previous Decade*			
		Births	Deaths	Natural Increase	Emigration
1930	1,543,013	39.3	22.1	17.2	2.6
1940	1,869,255	39.8	19.6	20.2	0.5
1950	2,210,703	40.7	14.5	26.2	8.8
1960	2,349,544	35.0	8.0	27.0	19.9

Source: José L. Vázquez Calzada, *La Población de Puerto Rico y su Trayectoria Histórica* (Rio Piedras: Escuela de Salud Pública, Universidad de Puerto Rico, 1978), pp. 12–14.
a. As of April 1 for each year.

In many branches of industry Fomento could provide employers with a female labor force that commanded a higher degree of manual dexterity than their counterparts in the States. These skills were an inheritance from the home needle trade industry that had flourished on the island during the thirties and forties. For many years, as a consequence, the majority of the jobs created in the factories that Fomento promoted were for women.[15] The entry of large numbers of women into the labor force inevitably contributed to important social, cultural, and demographic changes. The new role of women outside the home and their increasing importance as a source of economic support within the family were developments that profoundly affected women's attitudes. New attitudes coupled with new knowledge inevitably brought on new practices of procreation and family planning.

The creation of a middle class was another conspicuous consequence of Puerto Rico's economic development. Prior to World War II the island's income had been very unevenly distributed; while a relatively few families commanded great wealth, most subsisted in poverty.[16] With Operation Bootstrap a substantial proportion of the population, by virtue of increased earnings and greater educational opportunity, was able to establish itself between the very rich and the very poor. Although no narrowing of the extremes of income distribution occurred, the middle class swelled. Those who failed to gain entry into the middle class at least aspired to do so. An important feature of this was the adoption of middle-class values, and education emerged as a prime vehicle for raising one's social status. The acquisition of credentials became no less necessary to improve the employment opportunities of the young. More formal education, together with the much greater exposure of the population to the mass media, insured the increasing diffusion of the dominant attitudes and values of the society among all classes.

The intensification of the social and cultural interchange between Puerto Rico and the United States also increased this tendency. During the first four decades of this century, Puerto Rico was not only physically isolated but, because its population had but limited contact with the United States, also culturally remote and essentially self-contained. As suggested in a previous chapter, this situation began changing during the war, and was drastically altered with the postwar migration of Puerto Ricans to the United States. In contrast to the previous waves of European immigrants, the Puerto Ricans who came to New York and other American cities retained close contact with their island homes.[17] Many moved back and forth with frequency; they thereby shared at least a part of their new experiences with those who remained in Puerto Rico. Migration thus directly contributed to the rising tide of expectations that constituted both a major cause and a consequence of Puerto Rico's economic growth.

The intimacy of exchange was further reinforced by the influx of tourists and more permanent American residents and by the expansion in the workings of the mass media. Consultants from the mainland, no less than cultural transplants, reshaped popular expectations and encouraged a new sense of confidence about the future. For those involved in the development process, it was a time of excitement and enthusiasm; they combined high idealism with an optimistic faith that for every problem somewhere there was an expert who possessed the requisite solution.

In 1948, when the process of economic expansion was only beginning to take hold, Professor C. E. A. Winslow, a prominent figure in the public health movement in the States, visited the island. In an address to his Puerto Rican colleagues, he expressed the following vision: "There is an opportunity here to develop this island as the T.V.A. of the Tropics; not in the same sense, not with the same emphasis on power production, but with emphasis on intelligent long-range planning for the welfare of the human being concerned."[18]

The Tennessee Valley Authority, one of the more dramatic innovations of the New Deal, had inspired widespread attention as a vehicle for upgrading the socioeconomic conditions of a depressed region of the United States. Initially aimed at developing an integrated system of multipurpose dams, it had come to concentrate upon the generation of electricity. The characterization of the island's potential as "the T.V.A. of the tropics" was apt because the harnessing of human energy was visualized by Puerto Rico's leaders as the central thrust of Operation Bootstrap. Furthermore, Puerto Rico, like the TVA, was soon seized upon as a demonstration and a model to be emulated by others.

With the conclusion of World War II and the creation of the United Nations, the problem of assisting what were first identified as underdeveloped countries began to command increasing international concern. In 1949, shortly after President Truman established the Point Four goal of technical assistance to the less-developed regions of the world, Muñoz Marín offered Puerto Rico as a training ground.[19] Although Operation Bootstrap was just beginning to take off, the offer was accepted and the island was packaged and promoted as a "showcase of development."[20] In the face of the seemingly intractable developmental problems that many countries encountered, Puerto Rico appeared as a dramatic example of how an impoverished and stagnating population could almost overnight be reconstituted as a modern, relatively affluent, consumer-oriented society. As the Cold War heated up, the fact that this was being achieved by an American-sponsored political democracy that relied upon the workings of the free enterprise system did not escape attention. Modernization on the part of the developing world did not require the socialization of production which so many of the impoverished countries seemed intent upon pursuing: such was the message that Puerto Rico as a showcase appeared to proclaim.

There is no question that those concerned with facilitating development elsewhere in the world stood to learn much from Puerto Rico. None who visited the island could fail to be impressed with its rapid progress. Yet the transition to a modern, technically oriented society, with its accompanying affluence, was often made to look too easy. In a real sense, Puerto Rico's success was achieved not as a result of the enforced savings of its people but with credit spending. Escaping its agrarian past, it was reborn a consumer society, leapfrogging many of the long and painful steps assumed to be the requisites of development.

Here was a society which before World War II had been depicted as "the poorhouse of the Caribbean" aggressively aspiring to achieve the same level of per capita income as Mississippi, the target that was set by its economic planners. But because Puerto Rico's advance depended so heavily upon its relationship with the United States, the developmental strategy pursued by the managers of Operation Bootstrap could not be duplicated elsewhere.

The symbiotic but assymmetrical partnership between the island and the United States was consolidated in 1952, when Puerto Rico's political status vis-à-vis the mainland was formally revised. In that year the U.S. Congress conferred upon Puerto Rico a far greater measure of political autonomy than it had previously enjoyed. Puerto Rico secured the right to draft its own constitution, select its governor by popular election, and, within the framework created by federal legislation, exercise authority in all spheres except the military, the federal judiciary, and foreign affairs. Because Puerto Ricans continued to be citizens of the United States, they retained the right to unrestricted movement in all American territory. But because they had no voting representation in the U.S. Congress or the right to participate in national elections, they remained exempt from federal taxes levied against the individual. Thus, Puerto Rico became the recipient of most of the benefits and federal assistance which the federal government provides to the individual states, but it continued to escape most of the corresponding tax burden.

In retrospect, the designation of Puerto Rico's status as that of a "commonwealth" can be seen as an artful political compromise. It was tailored to the developmental course that had already been charted for the island. Among its virtues was its ambiguity. When the new legal instrument was rendered in English as a commonwealth, the American public encountered a term with at best uncertain connotations. To Puerto Ricans, however, the designation of the island as an *estado libre asociado*, literally a free associated state, suggested that it was no longer a U.S. territory.[21]

Most Puerto Ricans found the imagery of a free associated state attractive and actively supported the new relationship. It provided the people, long the victims of a sense of inferiority that had been the heritage of colonialism, with enhanced self-respect; this was important because of the traditional emphasis that the Puerto Rican culture places upon dignity. In the beginning few recognized how little freedom a free associated state might actually possess. However real the autonomy that Puerto Rico secured in local affairs, it soon became evident that the initiative for the future of the relationship was retained by the federal government. After 1952 Puerto Rico's leaders became increasingly involved in negotiating with the U.S. Congress about its inclusion in federal legislation and, when covered, in the programs of the federal agencies administering such enactments. At many points in the following years, the future of the island seemed to depend upon the effectiveness of its resident commissioner and its lobbying activities in Washington.

The creation of Puerto Rico as a commonwealth, nonetheless, helped greatly to harness the energy of the island in the battle of production. For more than half a century the issue of status had been a cancer infecting every tissue of the body politic.[22] The new arrangement did not prove capable of resolving the issue.[23] The society had for too long been polarized between advocates of independence and those of statehood to hope that the new status might constitute an ultimate solution. In the short run, however, it served to defuse the issue and push it into the background. It was a unifying force which moderated the disagreements created by long-standing differences. The increased authority that was granted to the island enabled it to act more decisively in domestic affairs and enhanced its power in dealing with Washington.

What it helped to achieve, however, also released forces that began to undermine the long-term acceptability of the commonwealth solution. As the movement of persons between the island and the States intensified, Puerto Rico became increasingly inundated with the mainland culture. When the mass media were not purveying U.S. imports, they presented unmodified imitations of the American product. Puerto Rico was by and large unable to resist this cultural assault except in those few corners of the island's new life where the traditional culture was fondly preserved, more as a tourist attraction than as a living entity. In addition, the expansion of the island's interaction with the United States introduced a variety of new and extremely vexing social problems. Drug addiction, juvenile delinquency, family disorganization, urban sprawl, traffic congestion, and other "social pathologies" were seen as the inescapable costs of this intercourse. Yet the society had little capacity to cope with such seemingly intractable problems, much less to resolve them.

Universally, these developments raised questions about the identity of the Puerto Rican society. The resulting identity crisis affected increasing segments of the population. The concern of Puerto Ricans to clarify their identity in their own minds inevitably revived a questioning of the island's legal and constitutional relationship with the United States. The issue of status once again began to provoke the same fervor and emotional intensity as it had commanded earlier. Puerto Rico's political leaders found that success no longer seemed to breed success; rather, it increasingly provoked uncertainty.

As early as 1955, in an address at Harvard University, Muñoz Marín eloquently expressed his own anxiety about the consequences of Puerto Rico's economic advance. With a poetical expression of concern for the future of his people, he called for the mounting of an Operación Serenidad as a counterpart to Operation Bootstrap.[24] Serenity, personal fulfillment, peace of mind—these, he suggested, were the ends that his society needed to realize; increases in people's incomes commanded significance only as means toward the attainment of these more ultimate goals. There was, however, no agency of the Puerto Rican government which was able to respond. No additional targets were set, no alternative programs were created, and no readily identifiable experts could be located in the new territory that the governor had charted. Operation Serenity became a cause of embarrassment, and was quickly forgotten.

The original brilliance of the strategy that guided Puerto Rico's postwar growth has faded in recent years, as some difficult remaining problems have been compounded. Today new uncertainties and increasingly deep ideological divisions convulse the island and tear at its fragile social fabric.

As a political commentator for the *San Juan Star* was to observe, Puerto Rico's history has moved "in spurts and jumps . . . not as the continuous flowing of the self-assured, but as the anguished tremor of the colonized."[25] Few societies have experienced such profound and rapid oscillations between hopefulness and despair. Dramatic improvements have taken place in the conditions of life of the Puerto Rican people, but no less important are the changes that have occurred in their opportunities, expectations, and confidence about the future.

The postwar years were years of hopefulness. Success in the battle of production, together with the substantial net out-migration during the decade of the fifties, relieved Puerto Rico's political leaders of the need to assert a clearly defined policy on population. Before World War II "overpopulation" had almost always been identified as either an insurmountable obstacle or a force threatening the island with perpetual impoverishment. The accomplishments of Operation Bootstrap suppressed, if they did not dispel, such views. They were inconsistent with the leadership's idea of people as the island's essential resource and its confidence that no problem was immune to solution through skillful social engineering.

The exuberance and optimism of the initial years of Operation Bootstrap unquestionably minimized the pressures upon Puerto Rico's political leaders to formulate a policy on population. Whatever their inner convictions, they were able to watch and wait and avoid taking a stand on this sensitive and emotion-charged issue. But the dramatic changes that occurred during this period also made people more receptive to family planning. The traditional resignation and fatalism of the society gave way to the conviction that persons could exercise a greater measure of control over the circumstances governing their lives. The importance of declining rates of mortality in this transition, particularly the precipitous decline in infant deaths, has already been emphasized. What had been an essentially frozen social order suddenly opened up for most segments of the population.

Important as these socioeconomic and cultural changes were, their effect on both policy toward and the practice of birth control continued to be filtered through two of the most pervasive features of this society, Catholicism and colonialism. The presence of the church and the continuing authority that Washington exercised over Puerto Rico constrained and obstructed the formulation of a public policy on population. And each in various different ways influenced the private decisions that persons made about the issue.

8. Turning Off the Faucet

Despite the hopefulness of the postwar years, many retained their anxieties about Puerto Rico's unchecked rate of population increase. Five births for every death, if not a certain prescription for disaster, necessarily jeopardized any chance that the island had to reduce its high level of unemployment.[1] Emigration was regarded as a temporary expedient, giving the island a breathing spell from the pressure for jobs.[2] As a stopgap measure, it was to be encouraged; as a more definite solution to Puerto Rico's "population problem," however, it was not acceptable. As Clarence Senior put it, relying on emigration would be like "bail[ing] out a wash tub while allowing water to pour in from a faucet."[3] The fundamental problem was therefore that of reducing the flow from the faucet.

With no official support from the governor or the commissioner of health, the government's family planning efforts were at a low ebb. The Health Department's annual report for fiscal year 1946–47 described a shift in the aims of the program and hence in its scope and efficacy.

> Our work was . . . curtailed in the year 1946 by a change in the policy of the Department of Health. . . . The name [of the contraceptive advisory service] was changed to Prematernal Health Clinics and it was specifically stated that these clinics would only have one determinate purpose: to improve the health of women. . . . Only in the presence of clear medical indications could contraceptive advice be given to these women. It was specifically decided that these clinics would have nothing to do with the problem of density of population. . . . This change in policy . . . has caused a great drop in the course of work. The number of passive and closed cases are constantly increasing. There is a lack of interest in the work by the Medical Officers, and also a deficiency in the follow-up work.[4]

Given this change of focus, those who had lobbied for policies to control population growth a decade earlier found themselves once again battling what they perceived as the indifference of key government officials. Those concerned with public health began to fear that the application of sanitary measures and the resultant improved survival rates of the Puerto Rican population were "acting as a sort of boomerang against the welfare of the island."[5]

In order to keep a close watch on population trends and influence public opinion in favor of birth control, the Population Association was created in October 1946. This study group built upon the interest generated by the Public Health Association's symposia on population issues, and, like its predecessor, was actively promoted by doctors Clarence Gamble and José Belaval.[6] Indeed, Gamble—as was his custom—sent medical statistician Christopher Tietze, of the National Committee on Maternal Health, to stir up interest in a prospective "action research" project and help set up the group. As a result, Tietze was named "stateside representative" for the Asociación de Estudios Poblacionales.[7]

Although the new association included as charter members many of the same persons who had participated in the Maternal and Child Health Association a decade earlier, the Population Association was primarily made up of university professors and government officials interested in demography and the social sciences. Assuming that opposition to birth control was rooted in ignorance or faulty interpretation of economic facts rather than in religious or moral values and that, once the facts were known, a growing number of persons would be converted to the cause of contraception, the new organization set out to gather and publicize demographic information. Through the publication of pamphlets and the sponsorship of forums and other educational activities, it tried to keep the public informed of the population issue in Puerto Rico. The association also sent reprints of articles on population control to heads of government agencies, legislators, and other influential policymakers on the island and obtained a subsidy from Fomento for the translation, publication, and mass distribution of articles on birth control.[8]

More important, the association profited by a general interest in demographic phenomena that prompted a variety of research projects in both New York and Puerto Rico. By 1946–47, Puerto Rico had become a laboratory for demographers and other social scientists, and the island's population had become the subject of much investigation, analysis, and conjecture.[9]

The Office of Puerto Rico in Washington commissioned the Bureau of

Applied Social Research of Columbia University to do a study of Puerto Rican migrants in New York City. The study was directed by C. Wright Mills of Columbia and Clarence Senior, who until then had headed the Social Science Research Center at the University of Puerto Rico. This project produced three kinds of information—demographic data on the migrants, welfare information on their needs for medical care and other types of social assistance, and psychological information on the migrants' adjustment to New York City—which was subsequently published as *The Puerto Rican Journey*.[10]

In New York the Welfare Council Committee on Puerto Ricans also studied the immigrants, stressing their needs and making suggestions for the better adjustment of the newcomers.[11] City College of New York also focused on the Puerto Rican population, supplementing and extending the Columbia project through research on community organization among the immigrants.[12]

On the island, research efforts concentrated both on the social factors leading to migration and on the fertility of the Puerto Rican population. Emilio Cofresí, a university professor with a particular interest in population problems, took a year's absence from teaching to devote himself to the work of the Population Association. During this time he wrote *Realidad Poblacional de Puerto Rico*, a brief in favor of a vigorous birth control program.[13]

The most ambitious population research effort was begun in 1947 by the Social Science Research Center of the University of Puerto Rico. The first in a series of studies was carried out in cooperation with the Office of Population Research at Princeton. This study, which used an island-wide sample of thirteen thousand persons, sought to document the cultural and social conditions affecting fertility and migration and to identify those factors subject to modification through public policy. The findings of the study, written by Paul Hatt and published as *Backgrounds of Human Fertility in Puerto Rico*, showed a pattern of high fertility among low-income families who had few years of education and poor housing.[14] One surprising revelation of the project was that a high proportion of Catholics favored small families and showed a minimum of religious objections to birth control. Hatt's research therefore posed the question, Why, if Puerto Ricans prefer small families and have no objections to fertility control, do they persist in having large families?[15]

In order to answer this question, the Social Science Research Center embarked on a more comprehensive four-year study. The first part of the research interviewed seventy-five families in an attempt to find hypotheses that would explain the discrepancy between small family ideals and large family practices. The result was *Family and Fertility in Puerto Rico: A Study of the Lower Income Group* by J. Mayone Stycos.[16]

The second part of the study used a sample of 888 families to test, quantify, and revise these hypotheses. This more extensive survey was carried out by Reuben Hill, J. Mayone Stycos, and Kurt W. Back.[17] It found that readiness for contraception varied as a function of three factors: favorable values, adequate family organization, and sufficient information.[18] Nevertheless, these were not sufficient by themselves to lead to the actual practice of birth control. To cross the line between readiness and action, a family had to recognize contraception as a salient issue.[19] In addition this study identified a number of cultural obstacles to effective communication between sexual partners. These included superstitious fears, modesty complexes, marital distrust, and lack of equality in marriage.

A field experiment aimed at increasing contraceptive use found pamphlets focusing on a limited number of topics more effective than group meetings.[20] On the basis of their findings the researchers described the existing birth control programs as "unsuccessful in making families systematic, regular, and efficient in their use of contraceptives."[21] They therefore suggested a number of measures to increase the proportion of the population attending birth control clinics, reduce the number of clinic defectors, enhance the use-effectiveness of contraceptive practices, and increase the ability of services to reach couples at an early stage in their marital histories.

Another noteworthy piece of research was that sponsored by Clarence Gamble. Its significance lay neither in its novel findings nor in its impact on public policy, but in the fact that its evolution was conditioned by the politics and practices of birth control over a period of more than ten years. As a result, this long-gestating project mirrored much of the social history of Puerto Rico between 1946 and 1957 and exemplified many of the population issues that were alternately highlighted and eclipsed during this period.

With the neglect of government-sponsored contraceptive services and the increasing importance being given to the study of population, it was almost inevitable that Gamble should rekindle his interest in Puerto Rico. As mentioned earlier, in 1946 he sent Christopher Tietze to the island on a preliminary expedition. The purposes of the visit were to "study the population problem, . . . secure the opinions of community leaders, and . . . determine local interest in, and available support for, an experiment in population control."[22]

Gamble's "intensive experiment" was relatively simple: it involved selecting a typical part of the island with approximately ten thousand persons and discovering whether it was possible to stabilize the population.[23] Nevertheless, the project required a preliminary testing of the political waters and the careful selection of a site with a large enough population to yield reliable results, a homogenous economy and culture, a predominantly rural character, and a cooperative cadre of health officials and community leaders.[24]

In order to probe the prevailing political attitudes concerning birth control, Tietze interviewed over twenty persons, including the recently appointed governor, Jesús T. Piñero, as well as Muñoz Marín and a number of other public officials in government and at the University of Puerto Rico.[25] Since Fernós Isern had vacated his position as commissioner of health and his temporary replacement was very sympathetic to the proposed experiment, Tietze was able to secure the support of the department in the experiment. The acting commissioner of health agreed to contribute medical personnel, contraceptive materials, and facilities to the project.[26] The chancellor of the university similarly endorsed the project and expressed his willingness to provide clerical support of at least two thousand dollars per year.[27]

Less tangible but more important assistance came from the politicians. Governor Piñero backed the project unconditionally and indicated that he would be ready to face the opposition if pressure were brought to bear to stop the distribution of contraceptive services.[28] Muñoz Marín also approved Tietze's proposal, but was considerably more circumspect about giving it his public support. His words to Tietze summarized his reluctance to alienate interest groups and his tendency to cloak potentially controversial views with euphemisms: "I am not afraid to fight anybody, but I prefer not to fight if it is not necessary. That's why I speak about the 'battle of production' instead of birth control, but what I mean is the same thing: a lack of equilibrium between population and resources."[29] Nevertheless, Muñoz explicitly approved the administrative assistance offered to this effort by the various government agencies.[30] Thus Muñoz established the policy of private support for and public disavowal of birth control, a policy which was to remain in effect for many years.

The selection of a suitable site for the project was relatively easy, since several of those interviewed by Tietze indicated a preference for the municipality of Naranjito, which had a high birthrate and met the requirements stipulated in the preliminary project design. In addition, the political and religious climate of Naranjito was considered to be favorable to the proposed experiment, and two of the three physicians practicing in the town indicated their willingness to work for the project on a part-time basis.[31]

Having done this extensive groundwork, Tietze reported to the National Committee on Maternal Health that most of the objectives of his visit to Puerto Rico had been accomplished.[32] Citing "intense and ardent support for the program" among the island's leaders, Gamble began raising funds and seeking other types of endorsement for the project.[33]

The optimism resulting from Tietze's visit, however, did not last very long. Tietze had left the island with the understanding that widespread sponsorship for the project had been secured and that Dr. Belaval would see the new commissioner of health as soon as he had been appointed to obtain his cooperation on the project. Dr. Juan A. Pons had been designated to the position in November 1946; by March 1947, Belaval had apparently not been able to see Pons, and both Gamble and Tietze were getting increasingly exasperated at this procrastination. Unable to get a report on the situation in Puerto Rico, Tietze wrote of the impossibility of undertaking the project without "a minimum of cooperation on the part of the organization in Puerto Rico."[34]

This apparently did not elicit much of a response, and Tietze returned to the island in November 1947 to find out what had happened since he had first obtained assurances of support. He discussed the question of sponsorship with Dr. Pons and with key university officials, who were all willing to go ahead with the project provided they were given a green light by the policymakers.[35] Tietze then went to see Muñoz Marín, who refused to do anything before the election and would not even allow him to continue with the preparations for the project because "there are no secrets in Puerto Rico." In Tietze's words, "He [Muñoz] was quite friendly about it, but . . . he was adamant."[36]

Muñoz's refusal to give public support to the cause of birth control was based on his reluctance to pay the political penalties of such an action. The 1948 election was a first for Puerto Rico: the Jones Act, which had governed the relationship between the United States and Puerto Rico since 1917, was amended in 1947 to give Puerto Ricans the right to elect their own governor. Muñoz Marín, leading the PDP ticket as candidate for governor, was therefore unwilling to risk his chance for victory by opposing those who rejected birth control on nationalistic or religious grounds. In addition, the Catholic church was a potential enemy of untested strength, and Muñoz felt personally vulnerable vis-à-vis the church.[37] He was divorced and had married a divorced woman after fathering two of her children out of wedlock. Any confrontation with the church hierarchy thus held the possibility of sinking from a discussion of ideological issues to the "politics of insult," with its attendant name-calling and muckraking.

With the project at a standstill in Puerto Rico for another year, Tietze and Gamble sought approval from the National Committee on Maternal Health, under whose aegis the project would be carried out and funded. In his request, Gamble emphasized the characteristics making Puerto Rico a particularly apt area for an experiment in population control: its high net reproduction rate ("greater . . . than that of almost any other country in the world"), the favorable political climate, the relative weakness of religious opposition, and the desire for contraception, which had been documented by several social scientists. He also argued that the committee's interest in solving Puerto Rico's population problem was "direct and immediate," since the Puerto Rican immigrants in New York represented "a drain on the city's medical services and relief funds."[38]

Pointing out that manufacturers of contraceptives and other sources had already contributed close to fourteen thousand dollars for the proposed experiment, Gamble obtained the committee's support.[39] His petition was granted in October 1948 on three conditions: that adequate funds were obtained; that the project was set up under the sponsorship of a continuing organization, such as a university or foundation; and that assurances were obtained that the project could be carried out with the continuing support of the Puerto Rican government.[40]

Confident that these requirements could be met, particularly after Muñoz Marín's electoral victory in 1948, Gamble and Tietze proceeded to recruit a field supervisor for the project. Carmen Rivera de Alvarado, who had long been active in the birth control movement and had served as executive secretary of the Maternal and Child Health Association, applied for the position, but was turned down. While admitting that her background, experience, and enthusiasm made her "a most desirable candidate for the position," Tietze and Gamble felt that her proindependence political leanings could "jeopardize the necessary good will and support of the Insular government"[41] and decided instead to select someone from the mainland, from whom they could expect "better preparation and training and higher standards of work."[42] This snub, however rationalized, eroded some of the support that Tietze had ably marshaled during his initial visit.

Public controversy also undermined official support for the project. In February 1949, *El Mundo* quoted Dr. Pons as having stated at a meeting of the Puerto Rico Public Health Association that he personally favored an intensive campaign for voluntary birth control and the use of district hospitals once or twice a week to perform fifty sterilizations per day.[43] A few days later, Pons had to declare that no official plan existed for performing sterilizations and that any decision concerning the implementation of such a program was not his responsibility.[44] Despite this clarification, Pons's remarks had caused an uproar and the governor's office issued a statement disassociating the health commissioner's comments from the government's official position. The governor's statement read as follows:

> It is not the policy of the government of Puerto Rico to solve the problem created by the imbalance between the resources and the population of the country by contraceptive means and much less by sterilization. Persons who express views to the contrary, though members of this government, speak strictly as private individuals. This government is trying to solve the discrepancy between resources and the number of inhabitants by means of the "battle of production."[45]

This incident, while effectively neutralized, made contraception a delicate topic and undoubtedly created a rift between the governor and his top health official.

Unaware of this episode, Tietze continued to press Governor Muñoz and Dr. Pons for concrete action on the Naranjito project. Meeting with no success, he wrote Estella Torres in June 1949 expressing his unhappiness and frustration and requesting her advice on the possibility of his going to Puerto Rico and "camping on the doorstep" until he obtained an appointment with the governor and the commissioner of health.[46]

They decided to pursue this course, although Tietze was not to be the one to "camp out" in Puerto Rico. By the fall of 1949 he had left the committee and consequently severed his relationship with the project. Dr. Wilson Wing, of the Johns Hopkins School of Hygiene, was chosen as Tietze's replacement. Thus it was Wing who went to Puerto Rico in November 1949 to find out what could be done to further the Naranjito project.[47]

After protracted discussions with the governor and Dr. Pons concerning the political hazards of population control, Wing was able to get them to approve the experiment once again.[48] They insisted upon a number of safeguards, however, to avoid even the suggestion of government cooperation in the project. First, the program was to appear to be only the routine activity of the Health Department when working with a full complement of health workers in one area, rather than the usual understaffed unit. Second, the importation of a mainland field supervisor, no matter how well trained and able, was vetoed. An outsider would only call attention to the project, thus attracting criticism. Third, women receiving contraceptive advice would have to have prior medical certification of need, although both "malnutrition" and "recent delivery of a child" were considered to be politically safe medical indications. Fourth, the choice of Naranjito as the site for the experiment had to be reconsidered: an energetic Irish priest had been assigned there since the municipality had first been selected, and he had apparently boosted the religious fervor of his parishioners. In addition, the news concerning the choice of Naranjito as a demonstration site had spread, and any increased health activities there would come under particular scrutiny and would be viewed with suspicion. Finally, all fanfare was to be avoided and no mention of the program was to be made, even in the States, to avoid the dangers of "grapevine telegraphy." Officially, therefore, the governor had neither met with Wing nor authorized a birth control demonstration project in Puerto Rico.[49]

Eager to appease all political sensitivities, Gamble and Wing agreed to the measures proposed by Muñoz and Pons and took even additional precautions. The project received the respectable title of the "Johns Hopkins Maternal and Child Health Demonstration," and Gamble wrote several sponsors stressing that *"no one* [be] *informed that there is a Birth Control experiment being carried on in Puerto Rico."*[50] Dr. Pons asked that all correspondence relating to contraceptive techniques or materials be marked confidential and that most letters be addressed to other members of the Health Department staff.[51] The project site was changed from Naranjito to Trujillo Alto, a municipality only twenty-five miles from San Juan but nonetheless still predominantly rural. These changes having been incorporated into both the study design and the unwritten code of population research in Puerto Rico, the project finally got started in March 1950.

In addition to the general goal of reducing the rate of population growth in Trujillo Alto, the project attempted to discover what method was most acceptable to the rural population of Puerto Rico and how instruction could best be given in a tropical area with low levels of education and per capita income.[52] The program design therefore included vigorous outreach, intensive promotion of contraception, and close monitoring and follow-up of both active clients and noncontraceptors. Additional physicians and nurses strengthened the services of the regular birth control clinic, and the project secured a jeep to facilitate the transportation of both health workers and patients. The contraceptive methods offered were Koromex cream, diaphragm and jelly, suppositories, Preceptin, condoms, and rhythm.[53]

Sterilization was to be recommended in cases in which there were medical indications, but the limited availability of hospital beds was a constraint on the performance of this procedure.[54] Nevertheless, this alternative was promoted by the opening of a hospital unit within the Trujillo Alto health center and the addition of "two young and enthusiastic doctors [who were] aware of the social need for sterilization in many of the women who come to the out-patient department" and who felt that "sterilization of the mother after the third live birth was a method of insuring better care for the children."[55]

A year after the project had been started, only approximately 280 cases were actively receiving services; 33 pregnancies had occurred among the study group. Home visits and follow-up on inactive cases revealed a trend toward sterilization, reaching 30 percent among program dropouts.[56] As the acceptance of sterilization rose, the relative emphasis given to this procedure also increased, with patient demand and availability of service mutually reinforcing each other.

The original project design also suffered other modifications as new situations arose and the possibility of meeting the stipulated objectives became more remote. By 1953, Wing was writing Gamble about the "gloomy picture" in Trujillo Alto, pointing out his disappointment at "the cautious attitude of all concerned, from the Governor down, which has made impossible any open health education campaign to promote birth control."[57] Wing therefore suggested reducing the number and scope of services provided while continuing the data-collection aspects of the project.[58]

Gamble, less easily discouraged, was not willing to give up on the experiment and proposed a different approach. Having concluded that there was "little hope of growth of population control under auspices which are entirely governmental," he recommended that the Population Association carry out the promotion for the project.[59] He argued that this group would not be inhibited by the political fears of the government and might be able to conduct a successful educational campaign.[60]

In the fall of 1953, Wing went to Puerto Rico to enlist the cooperation of the Population Association in the project.[61] This was accomplished, and in 1954 the study group reconstituted itself as the Asociación Puertorriqueña Pro Bienestar de la Familia (Family Planning Association of Puerto Rico) to provide contraceptive services, stimulate interest in family planning, and carry out research concerning the efficacy and acceptability of different birth control methods.[62]

By November 1954 the new set-up had been organized, and the project began testing the effectiveness of allowing a nurse to give birth control instruction and supplies to old or new patients in the home. When visiting homes, a nurse was under the direction of the medical director of the Family Planning Association, Dr. Edris Rice-Wray. At the maternal health clinics within the Trujillo Alto health center, however, the nurse became part of the regular staff of the Health Department.[63]

Under the sponsorship of the Family Planning Association the project offered a wider variety of methods and expedited the distribution of supplies. Closer monitoring of patients was also made possible. Thus Wing was able to write Gamble describing the revamped program:

> Since the climate of the health department is at present somewhat hostile to the birth control program, they are supplying routinely to their clinics only condoms, diaphragms and Preceptin. At Trujillo Alto . . . patients will continue to have a choice of the other preparations. . . . All forms of contraceptive material, with the exception of diaphragms, will be supplied by our nurse to patients in the home. . . . With new patients, the nurse will make a repeat visit in a month, but after that, intervals of two months will be the rule with adequate material given to cover the time between visits.[64]

In addition, the Family Planning Association employed a social service worker to visit homes on Saturday afternoons and Sundays, giving particular attention to those families where there was resistance to the practice of birth control on the part of the husband. The Social Science Research Center of the University of Puerto Rico also gave the project new energy, choosing Trujillo Alto as one of the sites for its experiment to determine what methods of health education were more effective in promoting the practice of contraception.[65]

Still, in subsequent months the project continued to be afflicted by the waxing and waning of Health Department initiatives, high staff turnover, lax supervision, erratic and inconsistent record keeping, and inadequate accounting procedures. Moreover, the Family Planning Association was becoming involved in other experimental efforts, and the Trujillo Alto project was beginning to compete unfavorably for the time and effort of the association's personnel.

In February 1956, Dr. Rice-Wray wrote Gamble to inform him that the Worcester Foundation had perfected an oral contraceptive tablet that was to be tested by the association clientele, and to ask Gamble if this method should be included among the methods offered in the Trujillo Alto project.[66] Gamble, who realized that the association was embarking on an important test which could result "in something much more acceptable and equally as effective as the vaginal methods," strongly counseled against combining the two projects, since "it would probably end all, or most of the testing of vaginal methods," thereby leaving their use-effectiveness in Puerto Rico undetermined.[67]

During the following year the Trujillo Alto project began tapering off, and the final process of data collection and analysis was completed. The researchers' central concern—to learn how best to provide birth control services to rural Puerto Rico—had been partially achieved. The Trujillo Alto population in the sample remained far from stabilized, but its fertility rate had been reduced: the unplanned pregnancy rate was found to be 42 pregnancies per 100 couples per year, approximately one-half the rate that presumably would have been obtained without contraception.[68]

After winding up the Trujillo Alto project in 1958, Gamble organized a survey on the use of contraceptives in Carraizo Alto, an area bordering the original Trujillo Alto site, to see whether information given out by the project nurses had spread to the neighboring communities.[69] By then, however, new contraceptive technologies had begun to command the attention of the birth controllers, and Gamble, like others, was eager to explore these innovative ways to turn off the population faucet.

9. An Answer to the Quest?

As most efforts aimed at increasing the practice of contraception proved disappointing, the advocates of birth control began to embrace technology as the answer to the population problem. A method that was safe, reliable, convenient, and aesthetic would, they hoped, overcome many of the objections associated with traditional contraceptives. To many birth controllers, an aspirinlike pill that would be unrelated to sexual intercourse and would "immunize" against pregnancy seemed to be the ideal method of birth control. By the early 1950s there were some indications that such a pill would be feasible. Advances in organic chemistry had made it possible to manufacture synthetic hormones, and biological experimentation suggested that mammalian fertility could be controlled by the hormonal manipulation of the egg's environment.

In March 1951, Margaret Sanger and Dr. Abraham Stone, of the Margaret Sanger Research Bureau in New York, met with Dr. Gregory Pincus to discuss the possibility of using steroids as contraceptives. Pincus, who had done pioneering research on mammalian sexual physiology and had founded the Worcester Foundation for Experimental Biology, agreed to undertake a research project aimed at developing a novel method of contraception.[1]

After this first meeting with Sanger and Stone, Pincus applied to the Planned Parenthood Federation of America for support of his proposed project, "Studies in Hormonal Contraception," for which he received a total of sixty-five hundred dollars in 1951 and 1952.[2] This modest sum provided Pincus and his associates with the financial aid required for the first stage of a more ambitious project.

The initial exploration, which was assigned to biologist Min-Chueh Chang, was based on the knowledge that progesterone could inhibit ovulation. Chang therefore believed that "one of the most attractive and promising approaches to development of an oral contraceptive was to investigate the effects of progesterone and the newly synthesized progestational compounds on reproduction by various routes of administration."[3] By April 1951 he had begun treating female rabbits with progesterone and related compounds by injection, feeding, or insertion into the vagina. The results of these trials showed that the administration of high doses of hormones inhibited ovulation, a finding that was subsequently confirmed in a second series of experiments conducted on rats.[4]

With these preliminary findings in hand, Pincus asked Albert L. Raymond, vice-president in charge of research and development at the G. D. Searle Company, to sponsor further investigation aimed at developing a contraceptive injection or pill. Raymond, however, was skeptical of the proposed project. Searle had already sponsored several other projects carried out by the Worcester Foundation, and the company felt it had received a scanty return on its investment.[5]

Sanger was more successful in obtaining the financing required by the scientists. In January 1952 she had met with Katherine Dexter McCormick to discuss the prospects of contraceptive research.[6] McCormick, a graduate of MIT whose husband was an heir to the fortune of Cyrus McCormick, had long been a champion of feminist causes, including suffrage for women and birth control. Having majored in biology, she had a scientific interest in the physiology of reproduction and was becoming increasingly impatient about the lack of a foolproof contraceptive.[7]

In March 1952, Sanger asked McCormick if she had heard about Pincus's research. She had not, and Sanger proceeded to bring her up to date on the developments in Worcester. McCormick and Sanger later met with Pincus, and McCormick agreed to sponsor the research that promised to free women from unwanted pregnancy.[8] From then on, McCormick became a committed supporter of the Worcester team.

The efforts carried out by Pincus and his associates were complemented by the research being conducted by Dr. John Rock, a Harvard gynecologist and director of the Free Hospital for Women in Boston. While Pincus and Chang were intent on suppressing ovulation, Rock was concerned with the opposite problem: inducing pregnancy in women with infertility problems. Rock hypothesized that because female sterility is often caused by subnormal uterine and Fallopian tube development, administration of sex hormones would "bring about a pseudopregnancy that would stimulate the growth of the tubes and the womb, correcting their dysfunction and making fertilization and pregnancy possible."[9] Rock was therefore administering estrogen and progesterone to a group of sterile women, and his hypothesis had been tentatively confirmed: out of eighty experimental subjects undergoing the treatment, thirteen became pregnant when the hormones were discontinued.[10] Rock therefore postulated that this "rebound effect" could provide a solution to infertility.[11] Nonetheless, the treatment had two major disadvantages. First, it was known that estrogen in massive doses could be carcinogenic.[12] Second, the treatment suppressed menstruation, and many women believed they were pregnant despite Rock's assurances to the contrary.[13]

In spite of their different missions, both Rock and Pincus were following similar approaches and were indeed working on different aspects of the same problem. Each had information and experience that the other could use, and a pooling of expertise and resources could be of mutual benefit. Thus, in April 1953, Pincus asked the research director of the Planned Parenthood Federation of America to approach Rock about cooperating in a study of progesterone as a contraceptive.[14] Rock agreed to collaborate, and the two researchers broadened their assays to include a wider variety of substances.

Following Pincus's suggestion, Rock began to experiment with progesterone alone (no estrogen) and instructed his patients to interrupt their medication after twenty days and not to resume taking the progesterone pills until the fifth day after their menstrual periods began.[15] This regimen met with success: ovulation was inhibited 85 percent of the time, and Rock's "rebound effect" was confirmed when four out of a group of twenty-seven women became pregnant within four months after terminating the treatment.[16]

Still, neither of the two researchers was completely satisfied with the results. Progesterone tended to cause "premature menses," or breakthrough bleeding, in approximately 20 percent of the cycles, an occurrence that disturbed the patients and worried Rock.[17] In addition, Pincus was concerned about the failure to inhibit ovulation in all the cases. Only large doses of orally administered progesterone could insure the suppression of ovulation, and these doses were expensive. The mass use of this regimen as a birth control method was thus seriously imperiled.[18]

Pincus began to search for a substitute for natural progesterone that would produce the desired effect at a smaller cost.[19] In September 1953 he asked the major hormone-producing companies for samples of the progesteronelike steroids that their chemists had synthesized.[20] The search for an oral contraceptive therefore proceeded along two tracks. In the laboratory close to two hundred compounds were being tested for their relative efficacy in preventing pregnancy in animals.[21] At the same time, the researchers were looking for possible ways to confirm their preliminary findings on a larger group of human subjects. In McCormick's words, it was necessary to find "a 'cage' of ovulating females" who would submit themselves to clinical experimentation.[22]

In February 1954, Pincus visited Puerto Rico. Although the main purpose of his trip was to lecture to the medical association and the medical school on the subject "Biological Synthesis and Metabolism of Steroid Hormones," Pincus took the opportunity to confer with a group of public health physicians about birth control on the island.[23] From his conversations, he concluded that the doctors were efficient and knowledgeable and that "work could be done in Puerto Rico on a relatively large scale."[24] Pincus was the guest in Puerto Rico of Dr. David Tyler, then head of the Department of Pharmacology at the University of Puerto Rico and an old associate; during World War II they had collaborated on studies of adrenal function fatigue and knew each other well.[25] Upon his return to the United States, Pincus discussed the situation with Dr. Rock, who agreed that as soon as they were confident of the indications of their results, they "should attempt in Puerto Rico certain experiments which would be difficult in this country."[26]

Writing to Margaret Sanger, Pincus summarized his findings to date and explained the nature and purpose of the proposed trials. The data he had accumulated were based on a dosage of three hundred milligrams of progesterone per day by mouth, and after two cycles some cases still showed no indication of the inhibition of ovulation. Further experimentation was required in order to manipulate the dosage and assure effective activity. The large-scale trials therefore involved "not tests of the contraceptive activity of progesterone, but tests of the effects of what might be the optimal dosage regime upon those phenomena which give us indication of ovulation."[27]

By the summer of 1954, Pincus and Tyler had begun planning a series of experiments to be carried out by the University of Puerto Rico School of Medicine. An "interested donor" (Katherine Dexter McCormick) was to make a research grant to the Worcester Foundation, which would in turn enter into a contract with the medical school for an investigation "of the effects of progesterone and related steroids on ovulation and related menstrual phenomena in women."[28] The research plan called for the administration by mouth or by injection of "suitable preparations" and the close monitoring of the experimental subjects by means of laboratory and other indicators.[29]

As originally planned, the joint venture between the Worcester Foundation and the medical school seemed mutually advantageous. As Pincus had indicated, large-scale clinical trials would have been practically impossible to carry out in the United States. Most states had Comstock-type laws among their statutes, as well as vigilant "bluenose brigades" who would oppose clinical contraceptive research.[30] Whatever site was chosen for the experiment had to meet two basic criteria: political feasibility and the availability of a collaborative team.[31] Pincus had found a favorable climate in Puerto Rico; government officials, hospital heads, and the dean of the medical school were all enthusiastic and helpful, and the mayor of San Juan had assured the scientist her full cooperation whenever he was ready to do active birth control work.[32] The second requirement—a willing and able research team—was also met. Pincus felt he could trust the physicians he had encountered in Puerto Rico because they were American trained and had "the American approach."[33] Moreover, he could keep in close touch with the program, since there were no barriers to communication.

In addition, Puerto Rico met a third, unstated criterion: its poverty and high population density provided a useful rationale for its selection as a testing ground. As one writer has indicated, the island was "crowded, impoverished and ripe for an intensive birth control program—a prototype underdeveloped country on America's own doorstep."[34]

For the medical school, the experiment promised nothing but bonuses: much-needed research dollars at a time when little clinical research was going on, the opportunity to collaborate with prestigious scientists, and the possibility of advancing medical knowledge. Those who had misgivings about being part of a program to develop an oral contraceptive could assuage their consciences: the project was labeled not as a study of contraception but rather as a study of the physiology of progesterone in women.[35] Despite the fact that McCormick's funding and Pincus's efforts were clearly oriented toward developing an effective means of birth control, the research could be justified as an end in itself, apart from its practical applications.

In spite of its auspicious beginnings, the experiment rapidly ran into difficulties. The first problem concerned staff turnover in the academic department under which the project was to have been conducted. Initially, the research was to have been carried out as part of the activities of the Cytology Center. The director of the center had therefore traveled to Worcester to meet with Pincus and Rock and discuss the details of the experimental procedures.[36] Less than two months later, however, he resigned, and the job of clinical investigator was reassigned to Dr. Celso Ramón García and the Department of Obstetrics and Gynecology.[37]

A more serious problem concerned the availability of subjects for experimentation. Although the members of the university faculty had expressed confidence that a suitable number of subjects could be obtained among patients, female students, social workers, and staff nurses, that proved harder once the actual experiments began. In March 1955, twenty-three female medical students were recruited; three months and four cycles later, only thirteen remained in the project. The large dropout rate was attributed to graduation and academic failure, misgivings about the experiment, and reluctance to adhere to the exacting requirements of the project.[38] Each subject was required to take her temperature every morning, take a daily vaginal smear on a special glass slide, collect a forty-eight-hour urine sample on a monthly basis, and submit to an endometrial biopsy once a month.[39] Even those who completed the four-cycle pilot study did not comply strictly with the demands of the experimental procedure. Some of the urine samples were twenty-four-hour collections, and Tyler wrote Pincus to complain about inadequate supervision and the lackadaisical attitude on the part of the subjects. Although these were "volunteers," Tyler indicated that he would hold accountable any medical student exhibiting irresponsibility in the course of the experiment, "hold[ing] it against her when considering grades."[40]

By the end of the summer the pilot experiment had begun to fizzle out. Dr. García had left Puerto Rico to work with Rock at the Free Hospital for Women, and his replacement was once again having difficulties obtaining suitable subjects for the study. Attempts to use the student nurses from the San Juan City Hospital failed completely. Although the director of the hospital and the supervisor of the nursing school had extended their full cooperation, not a single student volunteered to undergo the study. Only one medical student agreed to participate, and she soon dropped out. When private cases proved equally reluctant to collaborate, the researchers turned to female prisoners as a potential pool of subjects. Following a series of consultations with the secretary of justice and the director of the Women's Correctional Institute, the research staff moved its equipment to the prison and began setting up the experimental and control groups. Before long, however, the prisoners expressed objections to participation in the project and the correctional authorities withdrew their support of the research. The dean of the medical school met with physicians involved in the experiment and a review of the situation led them to conclude that the project would have to be dropped because of the inability to secure subjects.[41]

While the experiments with human subjects were suffering these setbacks, the laboratory aspects of the experiment were progressing steadily and yielding promising results. Out of the many synthetic progestational compounds ("progestins") that had been tested by Chang and his associates, Searle's norethynodrel and Syntex's norethindrone were found to be most effective for the prevention of pregnancy in animals by oral administration.[42] Pincus felt that these findings deserved publicizing, and in October 1955 he reported on the work in progress at the Fifth International Conference of the International Planned Parenthood Federation, held in Tokyo. After presenting the results of the animal tests using norethindrone and norethynodrel, he went on to state that the "delicately balanced sequential processes involved in normal mammalian reproduction" could be disrupted "in such a way that no physiological cost to the organism is involved."[43]

Pincus's language was vague enough to generate conflicting speculation. While some concluded that the attainment of an oral contraceptive was imminent, others felt differently. Sir Solly Zuckerman, who chaired the meeting at which Pincus presented his findings, was among the latter. In the late thirties he had been involved in research on sex hormones and had succeeded in demonstrating that the reproductive cycle of rats and mice could be suppressed by female hormones.[44] Yet he had doubts about the prospects of developing a contraceptive pill, pointing out that such a discovery was still "so remote from realization that ... no one [could] say how, when, or even whether success [would] ever be achieved."[45]

Rock was almost as guarded in his appraisal of the situation. Considering the animal experiments to be too tentative and inconclusive to warrant publicizing, he had refused to accompany Pincus to Tokyo and had urged his collaborator not to go.[46] In the fall of 1955, while Pincus was preparing his presentation, Rock was questioning whether progesterone was the answer they were all waiting for. One source of worry was the hormone's effect on menstruation: after prolonged dosage menstruation seemed to return, but with altered timing and flow. Another problem concerned the scientists' limited understanding of how the substance actually worked. In the words of Katherine Dexter McCormick, "The problem is that while we know that progesterone can and does stop ovulation, we do not know how it does it. If the metabolism of progesterone —its breakdown after it gets into the body, and its use there ...—could be determined, it may be possible to utilize it to the desired end, without bad effects."[47]

This gap in basic information in turn posed the moral question of how to achieve contraception without destroying life. Rock, a devout Catholic, was particularly intent on finding a solution that could be squared with Catholic ethics. The ideal answer required interrupting the reproductive process at the earliest possible stage. Without adequate information on how this could be done, Rock felt that "critical world problems" justified intervening between ovulation and the next menstrual period.[48]

By December 1955, however, Rock's enthusiasm matched that of Pincus: part of the scientific problem had been overcome, and the moral issue had been effectively postponed. The two synthetic compounds that had proven to be most dependable in stopping ovulation in animals and had shown the least interference with menstruation were tried on a limited number of women at the Free Hospital, and the results were "startlingly satisfactory."[49] Norethindrone (Syntex), administered in two daily dosages of ten milligrams each, appeared to inhibit ovulation without affecting menstruation or causing side effects. Norethynodrel (Searle) produced similar results. Rock was consequently satisfied that either compound was safe enough to use in field trials and, according to Katherine McCormick, indicated he would have "no hesitation in having them tried out to see whether they will prevent pregnancy in groups where other conditions (such as known fertility, adequate records, and general supervision) are favorable."[50]

In addition, Rock had found a way to set aside, if not solve, the moral question. Although the Catholic church forbade contraception through chemical means, no such ban applied to contraceptive experimentation. Rock therefore argued casuistically that clinical trials could be carried out *ex curiositata*. This meant that while he could not give a pill to prevent conception, he could give a pill to find out if it would prevent conception.[51] The Catholic doctor had thus found a theological loophole that allowed him to remain loyal to both his faith and his scientific mission.

By the end of 1955, Pincus was able to inform Tyler that the performance of one of the progesterone derivatives was "sufficiently well established to warrant direct trial as a contraceptive in a field study."[52] The substance chosen was Searle's norethynodrel, selected over its Syntex analogue (norethindrone) because in animal tests the latter gave signs of slightly increasing masculinity while inhibiting ovulation. Furthermore, Pincus had long been associated with Searle,[53] and the company was willing to supply adequate amounts of the substance for testing.[54]

Pincus wrote Tyler about the possibility of undertaking trials with this compound in Puerto Rico, suggesting that these be conducted through the birth control clinics and that Dr. Edris Rice-Wray be involved.[55] Rice-Wray was both medical director of the Family Planning Association and director of the training center at the Department of Health's public health unit in Río Piedras. Both jobs provided direct access to a pool of potential subjects, and she had indicated her willingness to cooperate in the clinical testing of new contraceptives when Pincus first visited Puerto Rico in 1954.[56] When efforts at the medical school proved disappointing, it was therefore logical for the researcher to enlist the collaboration of this hard-working, committed advocate of birth control.

On January 18, 1956, Pincus wrote Rice-Wray announcing a visit to San Juan, during which he hoped to confer with her and her colleagues "on the prospects of a trial with a new oral contraceptive."[57] The glimmer of success, however recent and limited, was apparently sufficient to erase the previous months of doubts and worries. Neglecting to state that the contraceptive pill had been tried on merely a handful of patients for only four months, Pincus was unconditionally positive concerning the experiences to date: these had involved small dosages and had produced uniformly good results and no observable side effects, and all subjects had promptly returned to normal fertility upon cessation of administration. He ended by saying that both he and Dr. Rock felt they had "an answer, if not *the* answer to [their] quest."[58]

Dr. Rice-Wray was very much interested in the tests and willing to cooperate. In February 1956, Pincus met with her and the clinical trials were set up. These were to be carried out under the aegis of the Family Planning Association.[59] Dr. Rice-Wray and Iris Rodríguez, a social worker, were to be in charge of the general fieldwork. This included recruiting cases, distributing the contraceptive, monitoring the subjects' reactions, and collecting the required data.[60] Pincus and Rock retained control over the research design and provided facilities for laboratory and other analyses that could not be done in Puerto Rico. The Worcester team also had responsibility for obtaining funds for the project, and they secured help from Searle and the Dazian Foundation.[61]

Because it had originally been anticipated that the subjects would be part of a rural resettlement scheme, the project had been cleared with the commonwealth secretary of agriculture and the director of social relations. According to Katherine McCormick, both were "quite willing to have the trials take place, but ask[ed] that it be done without publicity."[62] The site finally chosen for the study, however, was an urban housing development project in a slum clearance area in Río Piedras. This site was chosen because of its accessibility (no "wading in the mud," according to Dr. Rice-Wray) and the stability of its population.[63] A preliminary survey was made of young couples who had already had children (so that fertility had been established) and who intended to have more (so that a pregnancy would not be completely unwelcome).[64] The survey also gathered medical and menstrual data, screening out women who were over forty years of age or were otherwise unsuitable (for example, pregnant or sterilized). Those who were planning to leave the housing project were also excluded.[65]

By the end of March 1956, 100 women had been selected to form the experimental group. A control group of 125 was also chosen, both groups matched with respect to age, marital history, childbearing experience, and prior use of contraception. The experimental subjects were told that they would be participating in a birth control program; the women in the control group, that they were part of a survey on the size of the families living in the housing development. Both were informed that the effort was being sponsored by a private agency, unrelated to the government of Puerto Rico.[66]

The contraceptives were distributed early in April, and the women were advised to start taking the ten-milligram pills five days after the menses, whether they were bleeding or not. They were to take one tablet daily for twenty days, then stop. The need to follow the prescribed regime was stressed, since any pills missed would be likely to cause bleeding. They were further instructed that if this occurred, they should double the dose.[67] Despite the relatively complicated instructions and the need to take the pill every day, Rice-Wray and Rodríguez experienced no problems with acceptance; indeed, Rice-Wray reported that the patients were "crazy to get the pill."[68]

Less than three weeks later, however, the experiment ran into difficulties. A reporter from one of the local newspapers called the secretary of health, Dr. Pons, and questioned him concerning a program of giving contraceptive tablets to people in Río Piedras. Pons then called Rice-Wray, who told him that such a program was in progress and that she was directing it on her own time, apart from her public health duties. Although he replied that he did not see how the two could be separated and asked numerous questions concerning the project, he was finally satisfied that none of the patients was being examined in the facilities of the Health Department and that no public health personnel were working on the project on government time. These assurances did not conclude the matter, however. The following day the newspaper stated that Dr. Rice-Wray had "confessed" to directing the project and quoted Dr. Pons as saying that it was a "bad combination" for government employees to participate in a neo-Malthusian campaign. He also condemned the use of the Health Department as "bait" for the contraceptive program of a private agency.[69]

Dr. Rice-Wray never found out if Pons had actually made the statements attributed to him; however, she felt confident that the article would not harm the project. Nevertheless, when the social worker made a follow-up visit to the subjects, she found that "several women had stopped taking the pill, others had given it away, and several had doubts in relation to the effects of the pill."[70] Still, there were more potential subjects than could be adequately incorporated into the experiment. As Rodríguez wrote Pincus, women were continuously ringing up the FPA office asking for the pill, going to see Dr. Rice-Wray, and calling on her when she made the rounds of home visits.[71] As a result, those who left the project were readily replaced.

Besides adverse publicity, the onset of side effects prompted several women to withdraw. The pill's "blunderbuss" effect produced a variety of reactions. Some cases complained of nausea, dizziness, headache, and vomiting and refused to go on with the program. Others withdrew for different reasons: one lost her husband, two were sterilized, and several patients found that they were already pregnant when they began the program. By June, thirty out of the original group of one hundred subjects had left the project.[72]

Pincus attributed the side effects to the small amount of estrogen that occurred in the progestin as a contaminant.[73] The Searle Company therefore proceeded to synthesize a compound that would be free of the "rather potent estrogen" and advised Dr. Rice-Wray that future dosages would have less than 1 percent of this "impurity."[74] Subsequently, however, the researchers found that the pure steroid tended to increase the incidence of breakthrough bleeding, and the estrogen was deliberately included in the contraceptive preparation.[75] This was given the trade name "Enovid," consisting of Searle's norethynodrel with 1.5 percent mestranol as the estrogenic compound.[76]

In the fall of 1956, Pincus and the director for medical research at Searle went to Puerto Rico to supervise the field trials. The latter was impressed with the progress that had been made and guaranteed that medication would be furnished for at least one additional year.[77] Rock, however, still harbored doubts about the pill. While the substances tested seemed definitely capable of preventing ovulation, he had reservations about their being satisfactory oral contraceptives. These reservations were based on the possibility either that they might eventually cause permanent diminution of ova production, and hence produce permanent sterility, or that they might result in long-term damage to the endometrium. Rock therefore felt that additional substances should be developed and believed that the solution to the problem of developing a safe oral contraceptive would require intervening in a chemical pathway other than that inhibiting ovulation.[78]

Nine months after the trials had begun, Edris Rice-Wray resigned from the Health Department, where her activities were causing "much discomfort" to the secretary of health, and made plans to leave Puerto Rico.[79] Before leaving, she tabulated the available data and summarized the clinical experiences with Enovid up to December 31, 1956. Some 221 women had taken the pill, adding up to a total of forty-seven patient-years. There had been seventeen pregnancies, none of which could be attributed to method failure. The drop-out rate exceeded 50 percent; pregnancies, reactions, and sterilizations accounted for almost three-fifths of all withdrawals. Seventeen percent had experienced negative side effects, with dizziness, nausea, and headaches the most frequently mentioned complaints. Rice-Wray's brief conclusion was that while Enovid gave 100 percent protection against pregnancy, it caused too many side effects to be acceptable generally.[80]

Rice-Wray's successor in the program, Dr. Manuel Paniagua, found that the proportion of subjects dropping out of the project diminished over time, decreasing from an initial average of ten to fifteen per month to only three or four.[81] As the relative number of "survivors" increased, more women took the pill for longer periods of time, thereby yielding better data.

The perennial problem of side effects prompted additional laboratory and clinical research. In Worcester the researchers began experimenting with new formulations that would lessen or prevent the feelings of dizziness and nausea reported by many subjects.[82] In San Juan, where the high incidence of unwanted reactions was attributed to the "emotional super-activity of Puerto Rican women," Paniagua and Pincus devised a three-way experiment to test which reactions were "genuine" and which psychogenic.[83] One small group of new subjects was given Enovid with the usual warnings that they might experience side effects. These women reported such side effects in 23 percent of their early cycles. A second group, which had been using other contraceptives, was instructed to take Enovid and informed about the possible reactions. Unknown to them and to those who were administering the medication, however, they had received placebo pills instead of the oral contraceptive. Among this group, reactions were reported for 17 percent of the cycles. The third group, composed of new subjects, received the real Enovid but no warning concerning side effects. These experienced reactions in only slightly over 6 percent of the cycles.[84] Although the experiment violated two basic tenets of informed consent in medical research—that subjects be given a full explanation of the nature, duration, and purpose of the study and a description of discomforts and risks—it succeeded in convincing the researchers that a large number of the side effects reported were entirely or partially psychological in origin, a result of the user's expectations and fears.[85]

As reports of the pill's efficacy spread, an increasing number of scientists became interested in conducting clinical trials of their own. Pincus and Rock received queries from Japan, Mexico, Haiti, and India, but they were loath to involve themselves in efforts that they could not supervise directly.[86] This situation changed in June 1957, when the Searle Company released Enovid for sale. Although the drug required a prescription and was marketed for miscarriages and menstrual disorders rather than for contraceptive use, physicians were presumably free to prescribe it for any purpose they considered valid.[87] Thus Pincus concluded that there was "no reason why other qualified persons might not undertake experimental work with the drug."[88]

Clarence Gamble, always alert to research opportunities in the contraceptive field, showed an interest in starting a trial of Enovid in another part of Puerto Rico. He therefore got in touch with the medical director of Ryder Memorial Hospital in Humacao to ask about his willingness to test the oral contraceptive.[89] Ryder had participated in the Gamble-sponsored activities of the Maternal and Child Health Association in 1937 and had conducted birth control clinics over the years. In 1956, at the hospital's request, Gamble had donated a cautery machine for performing sterilizations and paid for the training of a physician in the use of the machine.[90] Confident of the hospital's interest in contraception, he offered to pay for the costs of a trial aimed at expanding and confirming the results obtained by Rice-Wray and her associates. Ryder was eager to cooperate in the experiment, and the fieldwork was entrusted to Dr. Adaline Pendleton Satterthwaite, a medical missionary who had been working in Puerto Rico for five years.

The site chosen for the trial was an area called La Vega, described by Gamble as "the most impressive" slum district he had ever seen: crowded houses "with scarcely room between for a squeezed pedestrian," no latrines, and no sewers.[91] It was felt that these backcountry handicaps provided an interesting contrast to the original project, permitting an evaluation of the oral medication under rural conditions.

In January 1957, Gamble visited Humacao and organized the project with Dr. Satterthwaite. Ryder was to provide the base for the fieldwork, and Satterthwaite was to supply medical supervision, including initial and follow-up physical examinations, instructions, and treatment as needed. A social worker would visit the women in their homes, supply the contraceptive pills, and collect the required medical and social data. Searle would donate the Enovid, Gamble would underwrite most of the remaining expenditures, and the Population Studies Unit at the Harvard School of Public Health would analyze the statistics sent from Humacao.[92]

In April 1957 the study got underway with the recruitment of potential subjects. Although Satterthwaite was sure that they would be able to "collect a goodly number of women who could cooperate in the program," the women from La Vega showed considerable reluctance to participate in the experiment.[93] Only 56 out of a total of 175 visited—less than one third—accepted the medication, and even those who agreed to participate had difficulty following directions.[94] In addition, the poor housing conditions in La Vega made the area a natural target for slum-clearance efforts. The area was soon razed, and the families were relocated on scattered sites, making the tasks of outreach and follow-up more difficult.[95]

In order to overcome these difficulties, Satterthwaite suggested doing away with the geographical restrictions and using the women coming to the clinics requesting contraception. These were better motivated and therefore more likely to remain in the program and produce reliable results. Although Gamble at first objected to this type of selection, he finally agreed to let Satterthwaite undertake an experimental series among her regular patients. The Humacao trials thus had two series of human subjects: the P-series (for Dr. "Penny" Satterthwaite) and the R-series, for Noemí Rodríguez, the social worker in charge of home visits.[96]

Like their counterparts in Río Piedras, the Humacao cases experienced a high rate of side effects,[97] with breakthrough bleeding the most frequent complaint.[98] In addition, Satterthwaite found marked changes in the cervices of those who had been on the pill for at least six months. Those who had had a slight cervical erosion before starting the medication experienced a worsening of the condition over time.[99] Although Dr. García and the Worcester team did not attach much importance to this reaction, Satterthwaite was concerned about it and fretted about not being able to get photographs for the record, since, "whatever you call it, the cervix looks 'angry.'"[100]

Despite these problems, the Humacao project expanded very rapidly and soon surpassed the Río Piedras series in volume and complexity. By

March 1959, Dr. Satterthwaite had an active case load of 180 subjects in addition to her regular clinic load of 50 patients per day; Rodríguez, whose patients had to be visited at home, had 130 additional cases. This large case load allowed the Humacao trials to introduce variations in dosage and to compare reactions between groups and the effectiveness of different levels and combinations of substances. It also gave the clinical trials greater visibility, and hence greater exposure to attack.

In February and March 1959, a group of Catholic social workers sponsored three television programs on contraception. The first of these focused on the oral contraceptive and featured two professors from the medical school, an internist and a gynecologist. The latter, who had participated in the university-sponsored pilot project under Dr. Tyler, charged that contraceptives were injurious to a person's health and that the pill could cause cancer. Although the family planners knew that both physicians were "rabid [members of the] Knights of Columbus" and were using their medical authority to promote their religious convictions, they felt that the initial volley required a reply.[101] The Family Planning Association produced a program stating that none of the 854 women who had participated or were active in the experiments had had cancer, but the harm had been done, and several women dropped out of the project.[102]

Nevertheless, the number of women participating in the Humacao series continued to expand, the case load being limited only by the supplies that Searle was able to provide. By mid-1960, the Food and Drug Administration had approved Searle's claims for the long-term cyclic administration of Enovid as a contraceptive. This authorization was largely based on the data collected in the Puerto Rican series, which included thousands of treatment cycles but only 123 women who had taken the pill for twelve cycles or longer.[103] Although the approval was restricted to the ten-milligram tablet for a period of not more than twenty-four cycles, the pharmaceutical company wasted no time applying for the use of lower dosages and hoped to secure permission to extend the limit of cycles.[104] It therefore had a direct interest in the continuation and expansion of the Puerto Rico studies and increased the pills available to the Humacao series to cover a total of four hundred subjects.[105]

In January 1961, Dr. Satterthwaite was invited to New York to participate with Pincus and Dr. Alan Guttmacher, professor of obstetrics and gynecology at Columbia University, in a closed-circuit televised panel discussion on the contraceptive use of Enovid. This activity, sponsored by Searle, provided an opportunity to present the data that had been gathered over more than three years of clinical trials at Ryder, and Satterthwaite took pains to update and analyze the statistics on a total of 730 women of proven fertility. The data once again confirmed that the oral contraceptive was effective but not risk-free. No woman who had followed instructions had become pregnant while on Enovid, and user failures accounted for less than 1.9 pregnancies per 100 women-years of experience. Slightly over one half of all acceptors had discontinued taking the pill for a variety of reasons, the most frequent of these being the onset of side reactions. Fully 65 percent of all users had complained of nausea, gastralgia, headache, dizziness, or other symptoms, and in 23.8 percent of the cases these had been sufficiently severe to lead to withdrawal. A total of eight deaths had been reported among the experimental population.[106] Five of these were flood victims; the remaining three deaths had not been autopsied, but were ascribed to cardiovascular incidents.[107]

Although the data were hardly encouraging this conclusion, Pincus took advantage of the New York gathering to hold a press conference announcing that the pill suppressed cancer of the cervix. Thus the implication was that Enovid could be introduced as a prophylactic against cancer which incidentally also prevented pregnancy. Interpreting Pincus's grandstanding as a "publicity stunt . . . to tap sources of income that wouldn't give to research on a contraceptive," Satterthwaite was embarrassed by the incident and glad that she had not been dragged into it. Guttmacher was similarly vexed, and he walked out when he saw the way the press conference was going.[108] Indeed, Pincus's announcement was later found to be premature and based on faulty statistics; nevertheless, he managed to obtain a fifty-eight-thousand-dollar grant from the American Cancer Society to carry out a randomized clinical trial and test his hypothesis.[109]

By May 1961, Pincus and García were meeting with Paniagua and Satterthwaite to discuss the cancer project. Pincus had secured the assistance of Dr. David Rutstein of the Harvard School of Medicine to design the proposed trial, which would focus on women between the ages of thirty and thirty-nine. The original research protocol called for a sample of ten thousand women (evenly divided between an experimental and a control group), but both Paniagua and Satterthwaite felt the massive recruitment this would entail was not feasible. Instead, they agreed to a small pilot project of only two hundred cases.

While Satterthwaite feared that Pincus would "stop at nothing to prove his point," she felt Rutstein would "not be a part of anything which is not carefully designed and controlled in such a way as to have some significant report, either positive or negative."[110] Gamble shared her concerns, concurring that Pincus was "apt to disregard signs which disagree with his hypotheses."[111] In addition, Gamble was worried that the long-term patients, which Satterthwaite had so carefully monitored, would be sacrificed to a new project of uncertain value. Moreover, he and Satterthwaite were beginning to test Syntex's norethindrone (Norlutin) and getting data on the reaction rate of that steroid in comparison with Enovid, and he felt she would have little time and energy to devote to a third research project. Gamble therefore asked Satterthwaite to weigh the dangers of getting involved in the cancer study, but left the final decision to her.[112]

Satterthwaite decided not only to participate in the cancer project but to request that she be relieved of her clinical responsibilities at Ryder in order to devote herself full-time to contraceptive research. The hospital routine was becoming a "terrific drudgery" to her, and she decided that research was the area in which she could make the greatest contribution.[113]

By the end of 1961, Satterthwaite had phased out her hospital duties and was supervising three research projects. Gamble had approved a modest budget for her.[114] This, together with the financial and other aid provided by Pincus and the Puerto Rico Family Planning Association, gave Satterthwaite the time and autonomy to continue the research on the Enovid series and initiate the cancer and comparative studies.

As additional types of contraceptives became available, Satterthwaite incorporated an increasing number of variations and combinations into her projects. Nevertheless, she felt that Ryder did not appreciate her research activities and chafed at the lack of support offered by the institution and her colleagues. The members of the hospital staff, for their part, thought that the research efforts were unduly separated from the hospital work and that information on the projects had not been shared with them as fully as it might have been. Gamble, who valued Satterthwaite's scientific interest, her skill with patients, and her ability as a gynecologist as a "combination which is unequaled anywhere in the world," advised her to grit her teeth and "stand the psychological discomforts . . . and carry on for the sake of the mothers you see and the children and the fathers."[115] He also suggested that she integrate the research into the other hospital activities, since only Ryder could provide the patients required for a study of the long-term effects of the oral contraceptive.

In the summer of 1962, Dr. Satterthwaite returned from a two-week trip to South America to find that the hospital board had approved the continuation of her research activity for another year and recommended a closer relationship with the hospital. Not all the news was encouraging, however. In her absence what she termed the "thrombophlebitis furor" had hit the island when a prominent internist loudly attacked the Family Planning Association for sponsoring the Enovid studies.[116]

The possibility of a relationship between the contraceptive pill and the occurrence of a spontaneous clotting in blood vessels had first been raised late in 1961 in *Lancet*, when a British physician reported the case of a woman who had suffered a severe, though not fatal, pulmonary embolism while on the pill.[117] At the same time, Dr. Edward Tyler of Los Angeles, the brother of Dr. David Tyler, observed that two young women taking Enovid had been stricken with similar clots, and both had died.[118] By the summer of 1962 rumors concerning a possible link between the pill and thromboembolic disorders were spreading in medical circles.[119] Puerto Rico, which had the largest and oldest population of pill takers, was no exception. The physician who sounded the alarm reported three cases of thrombophlebitis in Enovid users among his private patients and demanded that an investigation be conducted by the Department of Health.[120]

Although the birth controllers tended to dismiss the physician's report as a combination of religious fanaticism and medical alarmism, the Health Department and the Medical Association appointed an investigative team and hearings were held. One of the findings of the investigation was that all three cases of thrombophlebitis involved women who had obtained Enovid without medical supervision. The major recommendation therefore concerned enforcing the law that prohibited the sale of the contraceptive without prescription, and little was said about the pill's risks or long-term effects.[121]

In the United States, in the wake of the thalidomide tragedy, concern over the pill similarly resulted in uneasiness followed by pacifying assurances. Searle, which had a file of 132 reports of thrombosis and embolism among pill users, called a conference in September 1962 to discuss the safety of Enovid.[122] The cases on file included eleven deaths, yet the conference was brief and perfunctory. At a one-day meeting chaired by Dr. Michael De Bakey the majority of the participants agreed that there was no available evidence to show that the pill increased the risk of blood clotting.[123]

In Puerto Rico the thrombophlebitis scare resulted in the withdrawal of six women from the Humacao trials. Satterthwaite, who was "hoarse from trying to calm the others and point out that . . . there is no causal relationship, ... that we've seen no cases, etc.," was apparently successful in maintaining her subjects and even in attracting new ones.[124] By 1963 she was juggling no less than six research projects covering over twenty-two hundred women.[125] These varied in sponsorship, contraceptive methods employed, types of pills used, dosages, and patient monitoring. The initial "cage of ovulating females" had increased in scale and complexity to become a virtual zoo.

In June 1963, Dr. Satterthwaite left Ryder to accept an appointment as research associate in the Department of Obstetrics and Gynecology at the University of Puerto Rico, where the clincial trials had begun almost a decade earlier. From San Juan she continued to supervise the studies at Ryder, while undertaking new projects in different parts of the island.[126]

Satterthwaite left Puerto Rico in 1966, thereby concluding a significant chapter in the history of birth control experimentation on the island. As a postscript, it should be pointed out that the "thrombophlebitis furor" was subsequently found to be more than an empty warning. In 1967—more than five years after the first alarm—a British Medical Research Council task force concluded that "there can be no reasonable doubt that some types of thromboembolic disorder are associated with the use of oral contraceptives,"[127] a finding that was subsequently confirmed in a Food and Drug Administration report.[128]

The cancer study, which followed more than ten thousand women over a period of seventeen years, ended with a whimper in 1978. The Ford Foundation invested more than five million dollars in this study after the American Cancer Society withdrew its support. The ultimate value of the results obtained are questionable, however, and Pincus's hypothesis concerning the protective function of the pill continues to be debated.[129]

More recently, the evaluation of the hazards of the oral contraceptive has shifted from the area of consumption to that of production. The Ortho Pharmaceutical Corporation, lured to Puerto Rico by Operation Bootstrap and the prospect of a local market, has been the object of epidemiological surveillance and employees' lawsuits. Workers in the oral contraceptive plant have been found to suffer from sexual changes as a result of their occupational exposure to estrogens in atmospheric dust. Following complaints of breast enlargement in male employees and menstrual disorders in female employees, an investigation confirmed the effects of the synthetic hormone and pointed out the need to establish occupational health standards for these substances in the air.[130] The contraceptive pill thus continues to pose questions, rather than provide answers.

10. More Technological Fixes

Even as the clinical trials of the pill were advancing, the search for alternative methods of contraception continued. The challenge was to find a method which, in addition to being safe and effective, was low priced, simple to use, and dispensable without prescription.[1]

Oral contraception undoubtedly represented a technological breakthrough, yet there remained the need to provide a variety of services to persons wanting to practice birth control. Although funds provided by Searle, the Dazian Foundation, and Katherine McCormick to the Puerto Rico Family Planning Association supported the clinical trials, the association needed additional financing to meet its operational expenditures and carry out its regular program. While it continued to prod the government to strengthen its family planning services and adopt population control as an overt public policy, the association was committed to meeting what it perceived as the pressing need for contraceptive services. It therefore actively sought out and courted potential donors who could help the cause.

One of these was Joseph Sunnen. A prototypical Horatio Alger hero, Sunnen was the son of a coal miner and was a grade-school dropout who had overcome, in the words of one biographer, "a series of handicaps, setbacks and obstacles that would have broken the hearts and spirits of lesser men."[2] An inventor, he had developed a variety of precision instruments, which he manufactured in the Sunnen Products Company of St. Louis, Missouri. In true storybook tradition, luck, pluck, and mechanical ingenuity had earned Sunnen over fifty patents and made him a millionaire. With increased affluence and leisure time, he began to travel all over the world, where he witnessed in many countries the suffering caused by poverty and malnutrition. He attributed these ills to excessive population growth, and he resolved to do something about what he saw as the root problem of so much misery.[3] In the thirties and forties he thus made financial grants to several family planning groups and spent much of his time increasing public awareness of the population problem.[4]

In spring of 1956, while Sunnen was visiting with friends in Puerto Rico, Edris Rice-Wray took him to see what she called "some of the worst homes in the rural area."[5] He had met Rice-Wray in New York at a meeting of the Planned Parenthood Federation of America, and she had turned out to be the daughter of a former friend. Naturally, this visit sparked Sunnen's interest in Puerto Rico, an interest that was further fanned by none other than Clarence Gamble.[6]

Although Sunnen advanced some funds to the Family Planning Association immediately, he decided to embark on a large-scale project only after the fledgling association had drawn up a development plan for its activities over a three-year period. The plan set forth the objectives of the "Sunnen project" as (1) advancing the welfare of Puerto Rico by reducing the birthrate; (2) furthering planned parenthood objectives elsewhere by demonstrating effective action in Puerto Rico; and (3) strengthening the Family Planning Association for continuous and able work.[7]

The project centered on the promotion of contraceptive measures. While sterilization was part of the project, its role was limited to "instances where the demand and need are urgent and cannot otherwise be met," and focused on the male population.[8] It was explicitly stated that the project would not further the demand for sterilization, which was deemed to be already "far in excess of the facilities available."[9]

The plan went on to define the project's purview and clientele (low-income groups not being reached by other means) and stressed the educational and service aspects of the project. Unlike the efforts of Pincus and his associates, the Sunnen project was to be "not a research or a pilot project but an action program with a minimum of records necessary."[10] The plan contemplated the eventual absorption of the project by commonwealth agencies and the development of a firm financial base of contributions. The conclusions of the research studies that had been undertaken by the Social Science Research Center served as a basis for the design of the educational aspect of the project. Slogans favorable to family planning were to be used to counter negative attitudes, and pamphlets were to be widely used, their content designed in accordance with the findings of Hill, Stycos, and Back.[11]

The plan adopted by the board of directors of the Family Planning Association on August 8, 1956, was accepted by a representative of Joseph Sunnen and the Sunnen Foundation on the same day. The latter agreed to grant three hundred thousand dollars over the course of three years with the stipulation that this amount "be free from tax claims by the United States."[12]

The increase in funds allowed the association to expand its activities considerably. This in turn required moving into new offices and recruiting an executive director. Although Sunnen had initially expressed a preference for a male director, the FPA board selected Celestina Zalduondo, a social worker who had worked as a researcher for the Puerto Rico Reconstruction Administration and was heading the Bureau of Public Welfare within the Health Department.

Because the FPA sought to promote contraception throughout the existing public agencies, it exerted political pressure at the state and local levels to insure that birth control services would be available to those asking for them.[13] The association was heartened in this effort by the designation of Dr. Guillermo Arbona to replace Dr. Pons as secretary of health in 1957.

Arbona was known to be a strong advocate of family planning and had been active in both the Population Association and the Family Planning Association. Prior to accepting the appointment as secretary of health he had requested an audience with Governor Muñoz Marín. One of the specific points that Arbona brought up was his interest in birth control and his previous activity in the association. Muñoz agreed that an active program should continue and increase, and felt that the private, nonpolitical FPA could most profitably function in the area of promotion and education. Thus the association would act as a "lightning rod" for any political bolts from the Catholic Church, and the government could remain above the fray.[14] The governor said that the Health Department should provide all services demanded by the public as a result of such education and promotion, and gave Arbona a free hand in this matter.

In practice, however, the free hand involved a great deal of sleight of hand and delicate maneuvering, since services had to be strengthened and expanded within the strictures imposed by the existing health system. The actual availability of family planning services varied greatly in different parts of the island and among different segments of the population. What prevailed in fact represented the exercise of "local option" on this matter. The provision of family planning services by the Health Department was left to the discretion of the medical directors of the local health centers. If they did not wish to become involved in such work, whatever their reasons, that was accepted as their prerogative. If they did, then the central level of the Health Department was ready and willing to assist local efforts and to enlist the participation of the association in the work carried on in that locality.

The complex relationship between the state and local levels dictated government's involvement in family planning activities. Administratively, the island of Puerto Rico is divided into seventy-eight municipalities. These local units of government are directed by locally elected officials. The scope of their authority is restricted, however. Most governmental functions are carried out by agencies that operate on an island-wide basis. Thus, police and fire protection, the public school system, highway maintenance and contruction, and even local planning and zoning responsibilities are not under the jurisdiction of the officials elected at the municipal levels. Island-wide public authorities for the generation and distribution of electricity, for water and sewage, for telephone service, and for the construction and management of local industrial estates further limit the potential rule of local government.

The municipalities have, however, traditionally been involved in the provision of social and charity medical assistance to their residents. Over the course of this century, this local system of *beneficencia* that was an inheritance from the days of Spanish rule has been greatly modified. Under the influence of United States administrative practices all specialized medical services, as well as all public health and welfare activities, were made the responsibility of island-wide governmental agencies. After World War II, the Health Department undertook to develop health centers at the local level, initiating a new stage in intergovernmental relations in the health field. These health centers combined three separate units under one roof: a public health unit, a welfare unit, and a hospital unit. The last was operated by the Health Department on a contractual basis with the municipality contributing to its cost. Municipalities that had previously lacked the financial capability to construct, staff, and operate an adequate hospital facility of their own welcomed this development.

In a few municipalities, however, the mayors successfully resisted this development, seeing in it a potential threat to the authority and influence they commanded in their towns. Barceloneta, Luquillo, and Guánica, among others, maintained their local hospitals under municipal auspices exclusively. In these cases the Family Planning Association provided funds for surgical sterilization and contraception directly to each municipality. This guaranteed the availability of services at the same time that it deflected the attacks of the Catholic church against the commonwealth government. In Barceloneta, for example, the priest hung a black flag over the church to protest the sterilizations being performed in the municipal hospital under the sponsorship of the FPA.[15]

In other localities the attitudes of the locally elected officials precluded any cooperation with the FPA. As a result, there were marked differences between communities in the availability of services rendered by the government. Such services were at the mercy of shortages of contraceptive materials, administrative inefficiency, negligence on the part of the staff, or inadequate supervision.

The FPA attempted to compensate for the geographical unevenness of family planning services by creating communication linkages throughout the island. Celestina Zalduondo felt that public indifference, Health Department apathy, and religious interference could be successfully overcome only by reaching out and getting to the people. Sunnen, however, believed that the project that he was sponsoring in Puerto Rico required new birth control technology. Concluding that the contraceptives available failed to reach lower-income persons not familiar with the idea of birth control, he decided to take on the challenge of developing a more acceptable alternative.[16] Returning to St. Louis following a trip to the island, he therefore began to contemplate alternative avenues for dealing with the problem.

Sunnen promoted the idea of an aerosol vaginal foam that would combine two types of protection in a single product: a shaving-cream type of foam would provide a physical barrier inhibiting impregnation, and a spermicidal agent would provide a chemical contraceptive.[17] Despite the misgivings of at least one of his associates about packaging an inexpensive product in one of the most expensive types of container,[18] Sunnen took his idea to the St. Louis College of Pharmacy, where a preliminary product was developed in sixty days.[19] Following various tests to increase the contraceptive's effectiveness, he arranged with the DuPont Laboratories to make some representative samples combining the cream spermicide with the aerosol technology. These were then sent to Dr. Abraham Stone, director of the Margaret Sanger Research Bureau in New York, for further analysis and testing.[20]

Between March and October 1958, the bureau put the foam, designated as "aerosol vaginal cream no. 33J" through spermicidal tests and both single-dose and twenty-one-day clinical trials.[21] Once the spermicidal efficacy was confirmed and the preparation was found to be acceptable and nonirritating, postcoital tests were carried out to determine the degree of spermicidal activity *in vivo* under controlled conditions.[22] The absence of motile spermatozoa in these tests further indicated the high spermicidal effectiveness of the product.[23] Impatient to begin manufacturing the foam, Sunnen began to acquire the personnel, facilities, and equipment with which to establish an aerosol laboratory in St. Louis. Within a year the product was being manufactured on a semiautomated line in the facilities of the Sunnen Products Company.[24]

With the clinical tests completed and the product already being manufactured, Sunnen was ready to introduce "Sanafoam" to the board of directors of the Puerto Rico Family Planning Association in the spring of 1958. Squirting the foam into the hands of the members of the board to demonstrate its thick consistency and vanishing-cream properties, he convinced them of the versatility and desirable qualities of his new product. As Zalduondo informed Gamble, "They have developed a system that makes it possible to have the syringe filled from either end, including through the knob of the plunger. You can fill the syringe with the plunger down and store it under the pillow. The lack of light will not then present difficulties. . . . I have the impression that women will find this product acceptable."[25]

Sunnen was not inclined to submit the product to further testing, for he was convinced of its efficacy and safety.[26] Gamble, however, was interested in conducting and financing a test of the new contraceptive in Puerto Rico.[27]

Toward the end of 1958 the Family Planning Association received its first shipment of the foam. This had been rebaptized with the trade name of "Emko," a coined word chosen because it had no special meaning, was easy to pronounce in several languages, and was not hard to remember.[28] In January 1959, the FPA began the nonmedical distribution of the aerosol foam. At the same time, Gamble and his collaborators began a controlled study of the use-effectiveness of the product.

The area chosen for the field experiment was one of the worst slum areas in San Juan, known as "Los Bravos de Boston." The foam was offered to 222 women of childbearing age, of whom 69 percent agreed to use it. There was no evidence that religious scruples conditioned acceptance of the product. The safety of the product was once again confirmed, since no objective evidence of irritation was found among the women examined. The efficacy of the method was also established: the pregnancy rate, which was 80 per 100 woman-years of exposure prior to the test, decreased to 29 during the time the method was used. The report of the Emko field trial therefore concluded that the foam was acceptable, safe, and effective and that "its simplicity was found to be of great advantage in a public health procedure."[29]

In November 1959 the FPA began a large-scale program combining the new technology with an innovative outreach approach. The mass distribution of Emko relied on volunteer workers throughout the island. For the purposes of the program, Puerto Rico was divided into twenty areas, each including three or four municipalities. Each area was under the charge of a full-time supervisor employed by the FPA. The area supervisors, who included both men and women and represented a variety of fields (for example, teaching, social work, and nursing), lived in the areas and were familiar with their social life. The criteria for their selection were their ability to deal with people, their conviction of the importance of birth control, and their readiness to face attacks by the opposition.

Following a short period of training in the central offices of the FPA, the area supervisors assumed their duties, which included recruiting volunteers to distribute the foam, supplying them with the Emko containers, and enlisting general community support.[30] The volunteer leaders who received instruction on contraceptive methods and distributed Emko free of charge had to "have the respect of the group they serve[d], believe in the program, and have a spirit of service."[31] They ranged "from chauffeurs to court marshalls to carpenters."[32] The volunteers were free to choose their own ways of getting people to use Emko; these included making house calls, holding group meetings, showing films, setting up storefront clinics, and even conducting business out of a Volkswagen bus.[33]

Shortly after the volunteer program was launched, nine hundred volunteers had been enlisted and nine thousand cases had been recruited.[34] By 1961 there were approximately fourteen hundred volunteers and twenty-two thousand women in the program.[35] The number of active cases eventually reached thirty-five thousand, and the Emko Company hailed the Puerto Rico program as "the largest single volunteer program in the world for mass distribution of birth control items and information to low income families."[36] According to FPA estimates, the program had acquainted more than one hundred thousand persons with the use of at least one method, Emko foam, and had reached an even wider audience through its educational activities.[37]

Despite this widespread distribution of contraceptive material, the birthrate did not decrease significantly. Between 1959 and 1962 it went down only from 32.3 to 31.3 per 1000 inhabitants. And even this decrease can be largely attributed to the reduction in the population at risk, the result of emigration.

By 1963 the Sunnen Foundation had decided to start withdrawing its financial support of the FPA's activities over the course of two years. This had totaled several million dollars during the previous eight years and represented the association's major source of funds. Although Celestina Zalduondo repeatedly attributed the termination of Sunnen's support to his disappointment over the commonwealth government's failure to assume responsibility for population control and strengthen its contraceptive services, the phasing out of this aid was in fact the result of more practical reasons. First of all, the Internal Revenue Service had challenged Sunnen's deduction of the expense of producing and supplying foam to the association as a business expense. This resulted in a substantial tax assessment against the company and brought to a halt the free distribution of Emko in Puerto Rico.[38] Second, Joseph Sunnen had come to realize that providing free contraceptives to people did not have a substantial impact on fertility. In the absence of other enabling and structural factors, contraceptive technology was not enough. According to S. G. Landfather, executive director of the Sunnen Foundation,

> He [Sunnen] made large amounts of Emko available through Interchurch Medical Assistance to various parts of the world and conducted many programs in specific areas of the United States. The results were always the same. People took the Emko but the discipline and motivation was not strong enough . . . to be effective. So his great dream of developing a contraceptive which would have a significant impact on the fertility rates of the world did not materialize. It became quite obvious that much more was necessary than a contraceptive of any kind. People must have some compelling reason which causes them to go to the trouble of preventing the birth of additional children.[39]

However unsuccessful in controlling population growth, Sunnen's venture proved to be a financial success. Faced with IRS action, he proceeded to establish the activities of the Emko Company as a commercial enterprise. Accordingly, any contributions of merchandise would be offset by the sale of the vaginal foam.[40] After running in the red for the first few years, the company began to show a profit, grossing $4.5 million in 1968 and exporting its products to a worldwide market.[41] Like many other missionaries, Sunnen had started out doing good and ended up doing well.

Through the sixties Puerto Rico continued to serve as a testing ground for new contraceptive techniques. The existing core of researchers working under private auspices, the apparent abundance and acquiescence of experimental subjects, and the willingness of government officials to "look the other way" created an environment in which experimentation prospered. In addition to oral contraceptives and Emko foam, intrauterine devices and Depo-Provera were tested in Puerto Rico during the course of the decade.

Intrauterine contraception, which had been alternately defended and discredited since the mid-1920s, was rediscovered in 1960. Inert plastic devices that reverted to their original shape inside the uterus facilitated insertion and increased the safety and reliability of the intrauterine method.

In the United States, Dr. Lazar C. Margulies designed an intrauterine device (IUD) in the shape of a coil, which could be inserted through the use of a tube and a plunger without dilating the cervical canal.[42] Unlike the contraceptive pill, the IUD, once in place, did not require sustained motivation or constant medical monitoring. It therefore promised protection against pregnancy without the cost and inconvenience of the pill.

In September 1961, Dr. Adaline P. Satterthwaite met with Dr. Margulies and researchers from the Population Council who were outlining a study on the "action mechanism of the intrauterine coil."[43] With the help of Clarence Gamble and the captive clientele at Ryder Memorial, Satterthwaite began inserting Margulies coils in November 1961.[44] Shortly thereafter, a new device designed by Dr. Jack Lippes became available; this consisted of a polyethylene rod molded into a double S, which became known as the Lippes loop.[45] By December 1961, Satterthwaite had added the loop to the experimental group to include women from two communities in the mountainous coffee country of the island.[46]

Initially, the IUDs were given to women who wanted "one-shot" protection, but did not qualify for sterilization according to the age and parity criteria established at Ryder Hospital, and to those who could not take the pills or who found them unacceptable because of their side effects. Once the IUD became known, however, women who began asking for it were included in the trials.[47] As the experiment proceeded, devices of different sizes, shapes, and materials were tested.

A preliminary report written five months after the clinical tests had begun revealed that the method was "highly effective and free of infection and serious hemorrhage and in most cases of pain."[48] A more complete report covered a period of almost three years and included a total of 1,531 primary insertions. The extended trial found that a large loop was "the most acceptable and effective [of the IUDs tested], with minimal complaints and complications referable to the device."[49] Accidental pregnancies occurred at a rate of 1.5 per 100 cases, while expulsions numbered 8.5 and removals for medical reasons, 7.5 per 100 cases. Among the problems encountered were excessive menses, spotting, and discomfort. Nevertheless, the researchers concluded that "from a public health viewpoint, intrauterine contraceptive devices, especially the large loops, offer a promising means of population control."[50]

The quest for the elusive "perfect" contraceptive next focused on a method of inhibiting ovulation through hormonal mechanisms similar to those of the oral pill, but given by injection. The "shot," as its sponsors hoped the new product would be called, contained medroxy progesterone acetate and was manufactured by the Upjohn Company as Depo-Provera.

In January 1968 a project carried out by the School of Public Health of the University of Puerto Rico began using the new drug on a group of one hundred women. These were given an intramuscular injection of Depo-Provera every six months, and subsequently monitored in order to test the method's efficacy, acceptability, and side effects.[51] Excessive bleeding and discomfort resulted in patient complaints and medical concern, and the experiment was terminated on the grounds of unacceptability.

By 1970 long-term safety studies in animals had revealed that Depo-Provera caused both benign and malignant mammary tumors in dogs.[52] Other serious side effects of the drug included congenital malformations in children exposed *in utero*, irregular bleeding disturbances, and delayed return to fertility and possible permanent infertility.[53] In 1970 the Food and Drug Administration withdrew oral products containing Depo-Provera and a closely related product from the market and required a warning on the label of the injection.[54] The contraceptive use of the drug was further restricted in 1973 and finally disapproved in 1978, when the FDA notified the Upjohn Company that the benefits of the drug for contraceptive purposes in the United States did not justify the risks.[55]

Because this decision does not impinge on the use of the drug outside the United States, it is widely available elsewhere. Indeed, at present it is approved by sixty-nine countries, manufactured in at least six, and distributed to forty-two by the International Planned Parenthood Federation.[56] As a result, an estimated 1.25 million women currently use the drug, and many foreign governments and family planning programs have requested the FDA to reverse its ban.[57] Since the present situation strongly suggests the existence of a contraceptive double standard, the matter has become a heated controversy involving reproductive freedom, contraceptive politics, and the "global reach" of pharmaceutical companies. As one writer has aptly observed, "More is at stake than the licensing of a particular drug; the Depo-Provera case represents a clash of political, social, and ethical values."[58]

11. *A Single Instance of Inconvenience*

The introduction of new contraceptives, no matter how effective they proved to be or how convincingly they were promoted, had to compete with a growing trend toward sterilization in Puerto Rico. Under the Emko program the Family Planning Association integrated its support of sterilization with the distribution of the spermicidal foam; the area supervisors therefore had the responsibility of screening applicants for sterilization and making the necessary arrangements for providing this service.[1] The testing of oral contraceptives and IUDs required prolonged use, and the need for a stable experimental population often took precedence over the particular desires of the persons involved. Thus, in many cases sterilization was discouraged or at least postponed. Nevertheless, for an increasing number of women sterilization was the ultimate choice, and many who dropped out of the clinical trials found this procedure a more desirable solution to the problem of fertility control.

Sterilization is the most effective form of birth control, but it is also the most drastic: it involves surgery, terminates fecundity irreversibly, and forecloses all future options concerning childbearing.[2] It may therefore be thought of as a last resort, a possibility relied upon only after all others have failed or proven unacceptable. The choice of sterilization by an increasing number of Puerto Rican women thus deserves further examination.

Although there is no evidence that the programs sponsored by the PRRA, the PRERA, and the Maternal and Child Health Association included sterilization among their services, there is some indication that female sterilization was practiced in Puerto Rico in the 1930s.[3] A 1939 study of 1,962 families seeking services in the Maternal and Child Health program found that 4.4 percent of the female contraceptors had stopped using the method prescribed because they were no longer exposed to the risk of pregnancy.[4] The specific reasons grouped under this general rubric included sterilization, separation from husband, and "other lack of exposure." Though it is impossible to determine how many of the women in this category were sterilized, this patient profile provides the first documentation of the use of sterilization in Puerto Rico. Moreover, the study indicated that 34 percent of a total of 223 women refusing to try the method prescribed gave "no exposure" as their reason for nonacceptance.[5] Of course, those sterilized are likely to have constituted a small fraction of this group, since they would have had little incentive to participate in a program aimed primarily at fertility control. Although the percentages involved are small, they nonetheless constitute the first empirical evidence concerning the incidence of sterilization among Puerto Rican women.

It is generally believed that Presbyterian Hospital was the first institution to provide this service, in part as a result of Dr. Belaval's longtime affiliation with its staff.[6] Since this was a highly reputable hospital located in one of San Juan's finest residential areas, the surgical procedure undoubtedly gained respectability and even a certain aura of prestige.

By 1941 Presbyterian Hospital had acquired equipment for female sterilization through cauterization, and the director of the department of obstetrics and gynecology was eager to try it out on several patients who wanted to be sterilized postpartum. The "state of the art" was such, however, that the procedure left open the possibility of a subsequent ectopic pregnancy, with a fertilized egg becoming implanted within a Fallopian tube. This possibility (and its attendant mortality risk) was not only cavalierly dismissed but actually welcomed as an opportunity for the practice of surgical skills. "There are those who object that there will be a lot of ectopics following the operation, but the more the merrier, for I shall be delighted to operate on all the ectopics that happen! That is the advantage of getting to do one's own surgery."[7]

Despite the attitude reflected in this statement, the sterilizations at Presbyterian Hospital were performed with a minimum of publicity and were therefore not subject to criticism.[8] As the practice became more widespread, however, it became the target of religious and political attacks.

In 1943 the opening of Castañer General Hospital in the island's mountainous interior added to the facilities available for sterilization. This hospital was operated by the Brethren Service Commission and staffed primarily by U.S. physicians on volunteer assignments under its auspices; it served a population of seventeen thousand. Shortly after it opened, it began a vigorous program of population control. Because standard contraceptive methods were considered unsuccessful, sterilization was actively promoted.[9]

In February 1945, after 250 operations had been done, the Castañer project and its sponsors were attacked by the bishop of Ponce, who claimed that "all the men and women in the vicinity" had been sterilized.[10] He made his charge that sterilization and other neo-Malthusian practices had taken root in Puerto Rico in a pastoral letter which was read in all the Catholic churches and published in *El Mundo*.[11] This proved to be an effective means of communication, and Castañer was swamped with women wanting to be sterilized.[12]

Because the attack also threatened the Health Department, the commissioner of health sent the "most Catholic doctor" on his staff to investigate what was going on in Castañer. The data on the procedures done up to then revealed that the women undergoing sterilization had a mean age of thirty-two and an average of six children each. All the operations were justified medically, and the hospital services were found to have complied with the laws enacted in 1937 and confirmed by Judge Cooper in 1939. The hospital thus received a clean bill of health.[13]

In addition to increasing the demand for sterilization, the publicity generated by the case brought Castañer unexpected legislative support. At the time of the attack the legislature was in session and a subsidy for Castañer was under debate. The director of the project went to San Juan to find out how the bishop's charge would affect the subsidy, and was told that now he was sure to get it. This proved to be true, and the sterilization program continued unabated. Some four hundred postpartum sterilizations were carried out during the first four years of the project, and Castañer became a mecca for women seeking *la operación*. In contrast, attempts to interest men in vasectomies met with no success. The staff at the hospital encountered much fear concerning the loss of sexual potency, and no men were sterilized.[14]

The initiatives taken by Presbyterian and Castañer Hospitals in encouraging and performing female sterilization were soon followed by similar efforts at the Health Department's five district hospitals. As contraceptive services were curtailed, the demand for surgical sterilization increased and the district hospitals began to try to meet the need. Between 1944 and 1946 the number of sterilizations carried out by these public institutions doubled, reaching approximately one thousand per year.[15] Municipal hospitals also provided the service, but kept no records of their operations.[16] Anecdotal evidence suggests that some mayors exercised direct control over a number of beds and that these were frequently used for sterilization. Access to this procedure thus became a political "plum," to be dispensed as a special favor.[17] By the time that Christopher Tietze visited the island in September 1946, he could therefore report that in several public and private hospitals postpartum sterilizations of multiparous women were being carried out "almost as a routine procedure."[18]

As this type of surgery became more prevalent, the criteria for deciding who could get sterilized were relaxed. At Presbyterian Hospital, where 263 sterilizations were done in 1945,[19] the policy of the hospital was to approve the operation if the woman had three living children.[20] The unofficial policy of the hospital was not to admit multiparae, even uncomplicated cases, if they did not submit to sterilization.[21] "Informed consent" consisted of a printed form, signed by the patient and her husband, stating that she had been "well advised of the medical reasons justifying the sterilization and of the physiological consequences thereof." The "medical reasons," however, appeared neither on the form nor in the case history.[22] In other institutions even this perfunctory attempt at informing the patient was omitted. As a result, there were cases of overzealous physicians sterilizing childless women, a practice that was condemned even by the advocates of birth control because it threatened to bring the whole matter into disrepute.[23]

The trend toward "planned sterility" noted by Tietze in an article published in 1947 elicited predictable comments from the Health Department, the Catholic church, and the medical profession.[24] While Dr. Belaval admitted that 3,373 women had been sterilized in district hospitals, he emphatically denied that this was the result of a deliberate effort on the part of the Health Department.[25] Instead he attributed the rising trend to an increase in the number of willing mothers and acquiescent surgeons who chose to exercise their medical discretion in favor of sterilization. Thus he explained the reliance on *la operación* as a series of individual decisions based on the merits of the particular case and protected by the privacy of the doctor-patient relationship. The bishop, however, viewed the trend as a symptom of growing moral laxity and placed the blame on "the ostensible defenders of the public's health who . . . attempt to solve Puerto Rico's economic problem by reducing the number of Puerto Ricans while leaving untouched the causes and sources of [the island's] economic misery."[26] The Medical Association limited itself to a discussion of the legality of the practice of sterilization, stating that a physician could feel free to carry out this procedure as long as the aim was to "save lives and promote the patients' health."[27]

The fragmentary data collected by Tietze were confirmed by the islandwide survey conducted by Hatt in 1947–48, which indicated that sterilization had become "a somewhat common mode of birth control in Puerto Rico" and that 6.6 percent of all ever-married women in the sample had been sterilized.[28] The prevalence of the operation was found to be higher among higher-income groups and urban residents.[29] Its effect on the island's overall fertility was found to be negligible: it was generally resorted to only after high multiparity, thus averting few further births.[30] Over one-fourth of the sterilized women expressed regret at having undergone the operation.[31]

Still, sterilization was advocated by mainland eugenists as the solution to Puerto Rico's "reckless overbreeding." In their book *Human Breeding and Survival* Guy Irving Burch, then director of the Population Reference Bureau, and Elmer Pendell, an economist associated with the American Eugenics Society, commented that sterilization, "this substitute for contraception involving only one instance of inconvenience," was particularly appropriate in China, India, and Puerto Rico.[32] In the same vein, a plan with the title "For Great Problems—Great Remedies" was drafted specifically for Puerto Rico. It outlined how the island's population growth might be *"drawn off, provided for, or suppressed"* and proposed measures for all three objectives.[33] Together they suggested how half a million births could be averted in less than a generation. Those proposals aimed at suppressing the population focused on the early sterilization of both males and females.

> Great emphasis should be put upon sterilization for people who find it expensive or difficult to buy contraceptive materials or hard to use them. Praise ought to be lavish for men who seek male sterilization. . . .[34]
>
> The encouragement of female sterilization at the end of the *second* confinement should be part of any press campaign. Women should be instructed in the use of magic words which justify sterilization: chronic malnutrition, epilepsy, tuberculosis, . . . markedly low intelligence, . . . hereditary deafness—in short, whatever physicians will accept as worthy justification of sterilization at a given time.[35]

The plan stressed the need to adopt a series of "minimum targets" to stabilize the population of Puerto Rico. These included no less than one thousand female and two thousand male sterilizations per month over a period of ten years.[36]

These targets were in fact not very distant from those proposed by Dr. Pons in 1949 (chapter 8);[37] however, as they were neither politically acceptable nor realistically attainable, they remained unadopted. Muñoz's reluctance to espouse an explicit policy of population control, coupled with eugenic and medical pressures favoring sterilization, resulted in public laissez-faire, private prodding, and an acceleration of the existing trend. By 1949 it was estimated that 17.8 percent of all hospital deliveries in both public and private institutions were followed by sterilization.[38] By 1950 over sixty-seven hundred women had been sterilized in district hospitals alone.[39]

The number of sterilizations also increased in private hospitals, which Dr. Belaval had described to Tietze as "having no ideological scruples" and being "interested in the money" to be made from sterilization.[40] Indeed, some small hospitals were established in the 1940s primarily to perform sterilizations.[41] Yet by the early 1950s the facilities available were insufficient to meet the growing demand. As Stycos has indicated, "People began flocking to public and private hospitals to have their children if delivery could be followed by sterilization. When one metropolitan hospital temporarily abandoned sterilization as a result of criticism, it soon found its wards almost empty. Charging from 60 to 90 dollars for delivery and sterilization, private hospitals cannot keep up with the demand."[42]

As the acceptance of sterilization grew, so did the religious opposition to birth control in general and surgical procedures in particular. In 1951 a lay Catholic group, the Union for the Defense of Natural Morality, was formed to agitate against those laws it considered a threat to the "natural rights" of the Puerto Rican population. The birth control legislation enacted in 1937 was a particularly vulnerable target, and the union took aim against the "so-called eugenic laws," which had given rise to "a government-sponsored genocidal campaign."[43]

Although Pons denied the existence of a public sterilization program and stressed the health rationale and voluntary nature of the services provided under government auspices, the Catholic group continued its attacks and presented its position before the constitutional convention that had been convened in 1951.[44] The union requested that both sterilization and the dissemination of contraceptive information be banned in the constitution being drafted and that the rights to procreate and to "preserve one's corporal integrity" be included within the proposed bill of rights.[45]

When neither request was granted, the union urged that the citizenry vote against the new constitution.[46] The constitution was approved by more than three-fourths of the voters, however, and the issue of "natural morality" would have been quickly forgotten had it not been revived in the electoral campaign of 1952.

Formed when the proindependence faction within the Popular Democratic party grew disenchanted with Muñoz Marín's espousal of continued association with the United States, the Puerto Rican Independence party (PIP) included within its membership a strong group of Catholics, who succeeded in injecting a religious note into the party platform. The prevalence of sterilization therefore became a campaign issue, and the president of the PIP accused Muñoz of carrying out an illegal program of mass sterilization.[47] This earned the PIP's candidate for governor the indirect endorsement of the Union for the Defense of Natural Morality, which repudiated all other candidates as "unworthy" of the Catholic vote.[48]

The Catholic church officially entered the fray when, a few days before the election, the bishop of Ponce condemned the PDP as a longtime "enemy of Catholic ideals" and denounced the party leadership as materialistic and amoral.[49] This accusation prompted a group of prominent Catholics to explain why they were going to vote for the PDP. In a full-page advertisement they stated that, while they were against the policies of the party concerning divorce, contraception, and sterilization, they were in favor of the PDP's accomplishments and programmatic efforts in the areas of development and social justice and therefore felt bound by conscience to support the party platform.[50] The majority of Puerto Rican Catholics apparently felt the same way, and Muñoz and the PDP were returned to power in 1952. Whatever its utility in obtaining press coverage, sterilization proved a weak issue on which to rally public opinion and attract votes.

Two surveys confirmed the increasing acceptance of the practice on the part of physicians and women. The first of these, carried out in June 1952 but published a year later, indicated that 80 percent of the 453 doctors who answered the questionnaire favored sterilization for health reasons; 66 percent were in favor of the operation for reasons of poverty; and 63 percent favored it when the woman already had more children than she desired. Among gynecologists, the percentage in favor of sterilization for health reasons was fully 95 percent. Those who favored it for reasons of poverty or on the patient's demand constituted 65 and 57 percent of the total, respectively.[51]

This inclination among those who wielded the scalpel, combined with the tendency to define health reasons in very broad terms, contributed to a rapidly rising rate of female sterilization. The second survey, one conducted by Hill, Stycos, and Back in 1953–54, found that 16.5 percent of all women in their sample had been sterilized and that about 40 percent of all women who had ever practiced contraception had relied on *la operación*.[52] The study mentioned, in addition to the influence of physicians, three factors as possible explanations for the rising "popularity" of female sterilization. These were the "communicability" of information on sterilization, the ineffectiveness of other methods and the dislike that many women had for them, and the prestige of the operation.

The survey data confirmed the communicability of knowledge of sterilization, indicating that this procedure was more widely known than any other method. Women also learned about it at an earlier date, and it was the only method known by a significant proportion of women before marriage. The researchers attributed this familiarity to word-of-mouth communication and speculated that "in a culture where discussion of sexual matters is highly circumscribed by modesty patterns, sterilization is the only method which can readily be discussed. It does not involve reference to the sexual act or to sexual organs."[53] Unlike the word *sterilization* with its connotations of gelding, the term *la operación* inferred a surgical intervention, thereby implying medical need. The medicalization of the procedure, both in language and in practice, thus transformed an intimate, taboo subject into an open, morally neutral topic. This facilitated discussion between spouses. "We have . . . suggested that there are communication problems between husband and wife on matters pertaining to birth control. Here, too, sterilization as a topic for conversation should be easier. Moreover, once it is accomplished, further discussion is unnecessary."[54]

The second factor mentioned by Hill et al. as accounting for the growing acceptance of sterilization—the ineffectiveness of other methods and women's dislike for them—was documented by the irregular use of birth control and the high failure rates registered among a large proportion of the population studied.[55] Undoubtedly, inadequate contraceptive technology and poor motivation reinforced each other, with many women giving up on child spacing and planned fertility control in favor of the one-time, sure, "quick-and-easy" solution provided by sterilization.[56]

The third factor, the prestige of the operation, was more a matter of conjecture than of empirical evidence.[57] Nevertheless, the higher prevalence of female sterilization among the better educated found by Hatt and the impressions gathered by Hill, Stycos, and Back suggested that the procedure gained acceptance among the more affluent and educated before it was adopted by the other classes.

Finally, some have suggested that the Catholic population found sterilization more acceptable than other contraceptive measures. Resort to *la operación* entailed a single violation of church doctrine, in contrast to the repeated "sinning" required by other methods.[58]

The trend toward sterilization gained further impetus in the mid-1950s, when the research-oriented Population Association evolved into the more activist Puerto Rico Family Planning Association. The revamped organization had as one of its main objectives "the distribution of contraceptive methods and the provision of financial assistance for the sterilization of men and women," for which it needed personnel and funds.[59] A nine-thousand-dollar loan secured from the Planned Parenthood Federation of America enabled the FPA to hire a few part-time nurses to distribute donated contraceptives (creams, jellies, and foam tablets) and subsidize a few operations, particularly vasectomies.[60]

The funds contributed by the Sunnen Foundation in 1956 greatly increased the number and variety of services offered by the association and provided the means with which to subsidize additional sterilizations. Between 1957 and 1965 the association sponsored over eleven thousand operations. Approximately eight thousand of these were female sterilizations; the remaining three thousand were vasectomies.[61] Arrangements were made with private doctors, clinics, and hospitals, who agreed to charge a "group rate" for the two procedures: seventy-five dollars for each female sterilization and fifteen dollars for each vasectomy.[62] Those qualifying for the operation had to meet the following standards: minimum age of twenty for women and twenty-five for men; at least three living children; emotional stability; a thorough understanding of the irreversibility of the procedure; and reasonable expectance of permanence of the union.[63]

Changes affecting the role of women in Puerto Rican society further spurred the use of contraception and the reliance on "planned sterility." During the 1950s employment in home needlework, which had already suffered in the late 1930s and early 1940s, went down dramatically, declining from 60,000 in April 1950 to 9,000 in April 1960.[64] Nevertheless, during the same period the number of jobs for women in the service and industrial sectors rose from 120,000 to 133,000; thus some of those who lost their jobs in needlework succeeded in finding employment elsewhere. As indicated previously, the plants promoted by Fomento were particularly instrumental in providing opportunities for women. Many of these were labor-intensive operations that manufactured textiles, apparel, and precision products, industries that were associated with the routine, discipline, and exacting nature of "women's work."[65] A disproportionate number of women found employment in the new plants, and by 1960 Fomento-promoted industries had created 17,000 more jobs for women than for men.[66]

This shift in the island's occupational patterns and in the traditional role of women affected fertility in a number of ways. First, as women became providers they also assumed a greater decision-making role within the family. Their concerns regarding childbearing were therefore more likely to be taken into account. Second, as women became wage earners they tended to become more conscious of the economic implications of having additional children, thus increasing their motivation to use contraception.

Third, continued employment and procreation increasingly came into conflict. This was particularly the case in Puerto Rico, given the island's surplus of labor; any relatively unskilled employee could be easily replaced. Indeed, one rumor that Fomento did little to squelch was that women who were sterilized had better chances of securing a job, since they would not require maternity leave.[67] The Spanish word for pregnant (*embarazada*) regained some of the meaning implicit in its etymological roots, as a pregnancy became a source of embarrassment to an employee.

Moreover, the shift from home to factory grouped many women in a single location, thereby easing the problem of communicating contraceptive information. Some employers used this natural opportunity to provide orientation on family planning. The Family Planning Association promoted its services in factories employing two hundred to three hundred women, who would have been difficult to reach individually. In a brochure, "The Advantages of In-Plant Family Planning Services," the FPA tried to convince manufacturers of the economic rationality of promoting contraception by indicating that each pregnancy averted represented a "saving" of $910.[68] Thus Fomento and the FPA not only influenced women's relative power, their motivations concerning fertility control, and their access to contraceptive information and services but also enlisted the industrialists' cooperation in checking population growth by stressing the conflict between reproduction and production. In an ironic twist, Puerto Rican women came to equate childbearing with the production process, and the phrase *cerrar la fábrica* (to close down the factory) became a metaphor for sterilization.

Given this supportive milieu, it is not surprising that the number of women relying on sterilization continued to climb. A survey carried out by Harriet Presser in 1965 found that roughly one-third of all Puerto Rican mothers between the ages of twenty and forty-nine were sterilized, a rate significantly higher than that of any other country.[69] The rapid diffusion of the practice was equally unprecedented, with the proportion of women sterilized doubling during the course of a decade.[70]

This quantitative change was accompanied by a shift in the prevalence of sterilization by class. Presser found that women who were moderately educated were most likely to become sterilized.[71] Those with less schooling tended to have less information and therefore less access to services; those with higher educational levels opted for other methods of contraception. The relationship between family income and sterilization reinforced that found between education and sterilization. The highest proportion of women sterilized was found among those with family incomes between

$3,000 and $3,999 per year.⁷² Working women were more likely to be sterilized than housewives, and urban residents were found to have a higher proportion sterilized than their rural counterparts.⁷³

Although Presser stressed that the demand for sterilization in Puerto Rico was a "grass-roots" phenomenon, the historical evidence indicates otherwise.⁷⁴ To a large extent, the initial wave of sterilizations was physician induced, externally funded, legally sanctioned, and politically accepted (though not promoted). After that, the operation became established medical practice, and women began to rely on it as an effective contraceptive method. The demand for sterilization rose, reaching a point beyond which the procedure was no longer taboo, and requests for *la operación* snowballed. While it is difficult to prove that the choice made by thousands of Puerto Rican women was not voluntary, it can nevertheless be argued that this choice was conditioned and constrained by the surrounding social framework.⁷⁵ Medical authority, eugenist ideology, *machismo*, restricted employment opportunities, and the lack of other birth control alternatives were all factors that limited women's options. Reliance on surgical sterilization can therefore be considered a sign of resignation rather than of liberation.

While sterilization became one more contraceptive tool in the medical armamentarium and a rite of passage for many women, abortion remained a criminal offense. As a result, its performance remained a back-street procedure, shrouded in secrecy and sidestepped by both physicians and politicians as a controversial issue. Nevertheless, the question of abortion had to be faced whenever there was a specific complaint or compelling evidence of its performance.

In his annual report for the year 1933–34 the medical director of the San Juan Maternity Hospital stated that at least 60 percent of all miscarriages treated by the hospital were the result of induced abortion.⁷⁶ Although in some cases it was possible to identify the agent used to produce the abortion, the self-protective impulse of the abortees, together with their loyalty toward their accomplices, made it practically impossible to secure evidence against the performers of the operation.

The victims of botched abortions were just the more visible part of the problem. Some determined women tried home remedies, such as violent exercise or lifting heavy objects, while others sought help from herbalists or pharmacists, who prescribed a variety of ineffectual "cures" ranging from harmless roots to dangerous poisons. Quinine, for example, was thought to be an abortifacient and was prescribed and sold as such. Indeed, the association between quinine and abortion was so widely believed that the PRERA-sponsored program for the control and treatment of malaria was criticized as being part of the agency's birth control effort.[77]

Although both Hatt and Cofresí found that induced abortion was of relatively little significance in Puerto Rico,[78] as early as 1948 a Ponce physician wrote of the existence of an abortion "racket" and concluded that the liberal indication of sterilization could be a "useful weapon in combatting criminal abortion."[79]

The survey carried out by Hill, Stycos, and Back in 1953–54 revealed that 4 percent of the mothers interviewed admitted having had one or more induced abortions. Incidence was higher among urban mothers and more frequent among those who had had experience with birth control.[80] This figure tended to understate the true prevalence of the procedure, however, since women were as reluctant to talk as the interviewers were to probe.

In 1955, Celestina Zalduondo, at the time director of the Health Department's Bureau of Public Welfare, stated that hundreds of criminal abortions were taking place every day and urged the implementation of an aggressive program to diffuse contraceptive knowledge and prevent unwanted pregnancies.[81] Although no data were advanced to support her allegation, subsequent comments by physicians in government practice tended to confirm her estimates. In 1958 more than five thousand abortions were done in hospitals. In one municipal hospital alone, the number of induced abortions was estimated at five hundred per year, indicating a rising trend.[82]

While physicians blamed "midwives with neither licenses nor consciences" for the increasing incidence of abortion,[83] some of their colleagues had found it profitable to include this operation among their medical services. Each of Puerto Rico's major cities had at least one "problem-solving" doctor, who could be counted on to be safe, efficient, and discreet. San Juan had several "abortion mills," which catered to a growing clientele. As more physicians entered the business, two distinct abortion markets developed: the poor relied on midwives, who generally charged between twenty and fifty dollars per procedure; the more affluent went to the medical abortionists, whose fees were considerably higher.[84]

In the early 1960s an inquiry into the prevalence of abortion in Puerto Rico revealed that certain medical establishments were serving an international clientele and selling more than one million dollars of services per year.[85] The expansion of their business was attributed to the breakdown in United States–Cuba relations, which diverted to Puerto Rico women from the mainland who had previously sought abortions in Cuba. The

"Havana weekend," in which women from the States were taken from the airport to an abortion clinic on Friday and back to the airport for a return flight on Monday, had become the "San Juan" weekend by 1963. With few modifications, the system operated as it had in Havana. Island physicians had contacts in New York to promote the service and make the necessary arrangements.[86] In some cases only the site of the clinic was different from that of pre-Castro Cuba; the doctors were the same, since some of the San Juan clinics were operated by exiled Cuban physicians who had merely transplanted part of their network to Puerto Rico.[87] The charge for the procedure alone was said to be three hundred dollars.[88] With other hospital expenditures and transportation, the "weekend" bill was likely to be twice that amount.

Unlike sterilization, abortion had no advocates or public defenders. The Family Planning Association denounced the practice, citing both health and moral reasons for its opposition. In a leaflet with a silhouette of a pregnant woman and the words "Thou shalt not kill" on the cover, the association expressed its commitment to combat abortion and provide birth control services as an alternative to unwanted pregnancy.[89] The group also indicated that responsibility for fighting abortion should be placed in the departments of Health and Education rather than with the police and the Justice Department.[90]

In the wake of press coverage and a public outcry against the abortion racket, the Health Department, the Medical Association, and the Justice Department initiated a plan in 1963 to dissuade potential clients and even to intercept those who were about to enter abortion clinics.[91] A year later, the legislature passed two laws against abortion. One required compulsory medical reporting of all abortions to the Department of Health; the other eliminated the proof of pregnancy that had been required in any prosecution for abortion.[92] Since neither measure was aimed at the root causes of the problem—women's need for effective contraception and the willingness of some to satisfy and profit from this need—the legislation did little to stop the practice of illegal abortion.

In 1967 the Medical Association estimated that the number of abortions carried out in Puerto Rico each year ranged between five thousand and ten thousand.[93] Many of those receiving abortions continued to be women from the United States who knew of Puerto Rico's reputation as an abortion haven. Indeed, many on the mainland had the impression that the procedure was legal on the island. The president of the Medical Association reported that whenever he attended medical meetings on the mainland, he was invariably approached by one or two physicians requesting information on where to get an abortion in Puerto Rico.[94]

Although the Medical Association offered a reward of ten thousand dollars to any person presenting evidence leading to the successful prosecution of a doctor on an abortion charge, no one was able to claim the reward. Four cases were tried, but they all resulted in acquittals. The Medical Association leadership was forced to conclude that the high volume of abortions performed in Puerto Rico had made skillful practitioners of the abortionists and that "when a job is well done, there is no one to complain."[95]

The abortionists were equally adept at outwitting the law and keeping one step ahead of its enforcers. On one occasion the police attempted to frame one of San Juan's most notorious physicians by sending a woman detective and a companion to request an abortion. The doctor, whose own network of information was apparently more effective than that of the police, became indignant at the request and called the enforcement officers to report the two "offenders." The police arrested the decoys, who spent a night in jail before proving their role in the entrapment scheme.[96] Protected by a system based on graft, blackmail, and a "conspiracy of silence" among members of the medical profession, the abortionists were thus able to continue their lucrative practice without serious interference.

Since much of the extortion involved in maintaining the abortion clinics depended on the illegality of the practice, a legislator introduced a bill in 1970 to permit abortion under certain circumstances. Although the bill was far from liberal and allowed for the medical termination of a pregnancy only in cases of rape, incest, or a threat to the health of the mother, it was harshly criticized by many politicians, members of the clergy, and civic groups.[97] A poll among the membership of the Medical Association found the majority to be opposed to the liberalization of the existing abortion law, and not a single political party endorsed the proposed legislation.[98] Although the governor declared that he would veto the bill if it was approved by the legislature,[99] a group of religious leaders representing several creeds organized a massive protest march against the bill.[100] Following this demonstration the proposed reform was effectively scuttled, and the abortion statute remained unamended.

In 1973, however, the United States Supreme Court decided that a woman's right to privacy included the right to terminate a pregnancy of up to six months. Although this ruling superseded the local statute, the constitutionality of Puerto Rico's abortion law was not tested until seven years later. In April 1980 the commonwealth Supreme Court decided that the existing Puerto Rican law, despite its restrictive intent, was in fact more permissive than the federal standard.[101] The local ruling interpreted the existing law as allowing the woman to have an abortion at any time during her pregnancy. As a result of this decision, abortion is no longer a legal issue in Puerto Rico. It remains, however, a subject for political and moral debate.

12. A Matter of Conscience

While contraceptive technology and practices advanced in spurts, the cumbersome machinery of policymaking moved only with glacial slowness. Ever fearful of Catholic opposition, the Puerto Rican government made only minor adjustments and incremental changes in the birth control services it made available to the population.

Prior to the 1952 and 1956 elections Catholic groups had issued statements condemning the PDP leadership for its sponsorship of contraception.[1] But the charges had been successfully neutralized or rebutted, and birth control and population policy had been defused as political issues. This situation changed dramatically in 1960, when church-state relations and the ethics of public policy emerged as the dominant issue in the electoral contest for the governorship of Puerto Rico. In a major confrontation between the Catholic church and the PDP, birth control formally entered the political arena and became a rallying point around which factions were formed and pressure groups coalesced.

The issue of church-state relations first came to the fore early in 1960, when a bill was introduced by José Luis Pesquera, a prominent Catholic layman who was then a representative of the Puerto Rican Independence party. The bill proposed setting aside one hour a week for the religious instruction of children attending public schools and providing state aid to religious schools. Although the Catholic clergy and lay groups exerted pressure in favor of the proposed legislation, the bill was tabled by the PDP-led legislature. Governor Muñoz expressed his opposition to the bill by indicating that while he favored religious instruction, he wanted it free from all government intervention. He also argued that the school day was already excessively short and therefore afforded ample time for extracurricular activities.[2]

Angered by these manifestations of legislative inaction and executive disapproval, the sponsors of the bill celebrated a mass meeting which was attended by an estimated sixty-five to one hundred thousand persons. The

Most Reverend James P. Davis, bishop of San Juan's Catholic diocese, addressed the gathering, telling them they were "free to organize themselves into a political party" and urging them not to support any anti-Catholic candidate for political office. Following the meeting, leaders of Catholic organizations were quoted as saying that the formation of a Catholic political party was "a concrete possibility" because none of the existing parties represented the religious sentiments of the majority of the Puerto Ricans.[3]

Shortly after the meeting, Bishop Davis declared that Catholics had lost confidence in the existing political parties because they had disregarded the majority's right to petition for legislation that reflected Christian morality. He also decried the enactment of laws that were inimical to Catholic values, citing the 1937 neo-Malthusian laws as an example.[4]

Given the bishop's blessing and an indication of popular support, a group of Catholic laymen organized the Christian Action party (CAP) and began a drive to register the party with the insular Board of Elections.[5] The new party's leadership was derived from university professors, lawyers, doctors, and other professionals, most of whom were actively involved in and identified with already existing political parties.[6] It was particularly nourished by Catholic members of the PIP and the Statehood Republican party (SRP), but included a sprinkling of dissident *populares*. The appeal of the new party was based almost exclusively on its support of religious instruction for public school pupils and its objection to existing legislation on birth control and sterilization.[7] United on these issues, the members of the CAP thus overcame their profound ideological differences concerning the political status of Puerto Rico.

Concerted support by the Catholic clergy facilitated the registration of the CAP by giving the party an organized network extending into every parish and Catholic school. In July 1960, bishops James P. Davis of San Juan and James E. McManus of Ponce issued a pastoral letter describing the CAP as "the answer to the intolerable attitude" of the island's established political parties and denouncing the latter for following a "materialistic" philosophy of government.[8] The bishops subsequently authorized the use of church property to assist in the registration of the new party.[9] Parochial school buses, for example, were used to transport CAP supporters to meetings, and Catholic schools became satellite party headquarters all over the island.

In a second pastoral letter, Bishop McManus said that every citizen had "the obligation in conscience to vote only . . . for those candidates who . . . will best promote the civil and religious interests of the people." He also defended the clergy's role in politics by indicating that "bishops and priests would not be worthy leaders if they remained with their arms crossed, leaving the believers to carry the weight and responsibilities of the enterprise."[10]

The two leading parties adopted different strategies toward this challenge. While Muñoz predicted that the PDP would garner 60 percent of the vote and dismissed the CAP as politically weak, he nevertheless vigorously opposed the party as representing a "tragic mixture of politics and religion" and "a grave danger to the country."[11]

The SRP was in a more difficult position. Although its leadership was predominantly Catholic and it welcomed the possibility of a united front against the PDP, it also knew that a new party could siphon off votes from its already precarious position as the largest minority party. Luis A. Ferré, the SRP's gubernatorial candidate, had therefore tried to persuade one of the bishops not to sponsor a new political party. As Ferré was to admit later, he was aware that such a party would "hurt [his] own candidacy, . . . hurt Puerto Rico, and . . . hurt the Church."[12]

The SRP's difficulties were further compounded by its ambiguous stance on the issue of birth control. The party had been responsible for the enactment of the 1937 laws governing contraception and compulsory sterilization; indeed, Miguel A. García Méndez, the SRP's president, had actively lobbied in favor of the legislation. Ferré, however, chided Muñoz for wanting "to make it as easy to get sterilized as to eat an ice cream"[13] and condemned sterilization as "highly detrimental to the emotional stability and the health of the individual."[14] This disparity of views was eventually resolved when the SRP decided to co-opt the CAP by adopting in its own platform two of the CAP's key planks. The Republican party therefore supported religious education for the island's school children and promised to amend the existing birth control legislation.[15]

By then, however, the CAP was an officially registered party growing in both strength and stridency. By August, even Muñoz Marín had begun to give the new party serious consideration. Worried about the increasing number of CAP flags flying from the rooftops of Puerto Rico's barrios, Muñoz took to the campaign trail with the CAP as his main campaign issue. In his speeches, the governor repeatedly hammered at three themes. The first was that being a good *popular* was not incompatible with being a good Catholic. The second theme was that "when the clergy talk politics they talk as citizens." Muñoz therefore stressed that Catholics were not obligated to follow the clergy's political advice as they would be obligated to follow their religious counsel. In his third point, Muñoz held up the history of other Latin countries as proof of the danger of mixing religion and politics.[16]

A month before the election the political controversy was heightened when Francis Cardinal Spellman of New York visited Puerto Rico. Although the official purpose of his visit was to preside over the installation of Bishop Davis as archbishop of San Juan and to officiate at the consecration of a Puerto Rican, Luis Aponte Martínez, as auxiliary bishop of Ponce, Spellman had ample opportunity to acquaint himself with the local political situation. A group of prominent Catholic *populares* was on hand to welcome the cardinal, who subsequently accepted an invitation to have lunch with Muñoz. After meeting with the governor, Spellman was asked to comment on the bishops' involvement in the CAP. Spellman's diplomatic reply was, "I keep out of politics. It is outside my competence and will,"[17] thereby implying that Davis and McManus should do the same.

Scarcely a week later, however, the bishops further escalated the conflict by issuing a pastoral letter prohibiting the Catholics of Puerto Rico from voting for Muñoz Marín and the PDP. Citing doctrinal grounds for their ban, the bishops particularly condemned a portion of the PDP platform as heretical. The focus for episcopal concern was a paragraph suggesting that majority opinion was the determining principle in defining public morality. The actual text of the PDP platform read as follows: "The democratic philosophy of our Party implies that sanctions can be used to prohibit those acts which the general consensus of Puerto Rican opinion considers immoral . . . but in a free society, it is not legal to forbid by sanctions those acts which a respectable portion of public opinion does not consider to be immoral."[18] Decrying this doctrine of moral relativism, the bishops concluded it was their obligation "to prohibit Catholics from giving their votes to a party that accepts as its own the morality of 'the regime of liberty' negating Christian principles."[19]

The anti-PDP letter was read at all the masses, causing great political turmoil throughout the island and beyond. Inés Mendoza de Muñoz, the governor's wife, walked out of the mass and was promptly followed by a group of loyal *populares*. The moment was captured by a photographer from *Life*, and Puerto Rico instantly became a newsworthy subject for members of the international press and cameramen from the major U.S. television networks.[20]

The political fallout from these events reached the mainland almost immediately. John F. Kennedy, who aspired to become his country's first Catholic president, quickly reacted to the pastoral letter, calling the bishops' action "wholly improper" and disagreeing with the right of the Puerto Rican clergy to instruct parishioners how to vote. Muñoz sent a trusted emissary to meet with Robert F. Kennedy, then serving as his brother's campaign manager. Muñoz sought to counteract the bishops' accusations, while the Kennedys attempted to quarantine the Puerto Rican dispute. Subsequent declarations of several distinguished Catholic prelates accomplished both aims.

Cardinal Spellman said that Roman Catholic voters in Puerto Rico would not be committing a sin, nor would they be penalized by the church, if they voted contrary to a directive issued by the Puerto Rican bishops. He also indicated that the issue at hand was a matter between Catholics and their consciences.[21] Other members of the clergy emphasized the distinctive nature of the Puerto Rican case and dismissed the possibility of any similar conflict occurring in the United States.

The personal representative of Pope John XXIII in the United States said he was confident that the Roman Catholic hierarchy in the United States would never engage in political action similar to that of the Puerto Rican bishops.[22] Expanding on the same theme, Richard Cardinal Cushing of Boston stated it was "totally out of step with the American tradition" for ecclesiastical authority to dictate political voting. "This has never been part of our history, and I pray God that it never will be." Cushing then went on to define the subtle boundary between legitimate ministerial guidance and political interference.

> We expect religious leaders in our country of whatever denomination to discuss those issues which have relevance to public order and to advise their constituents when spiritual principles and religious values are involved. This is not improperly mixing religion and politics; this is bringing our religious traditions into the stream of American life in a way that influences that public life while it protects individual freedom. . . . However, . . . the American tradition . . . is satisfied simply to call to public attention moral questions with their implications and leave to the conscience of the people the specific political decision which comes in the act of voting.[23]

Muñoz also emphasized this last theme, labeling the bishops' actions "anti–Puerto Rican, anti-American and anti-democratic."[24] This message was carried throughout the island as part of a "Victory Caravan," in which Muñoz visited every town, delivering between ten and twelve speeches per day. Confronted by the anguish of many Catholic *populares*, he lashed at the bishops' ban, characterizing it as a throwback to "medieval obscurantism" and "an incredible and unjust intervention in the rights and political freedom of the citizens of Puerto Rico."[25]

The bishops, however, insisted that the PDP had substituted the will of the people for the authority of God and continued to defend their right to use their spiritual authority to influence the Catholic vote.[26] Indeed, their position became increasingly rigid over time. In yet another pastoral letter, this one read in all of the island's Catholic churches just ten days before the election, they stated that voting for the PDP was a sin. Unlike their previous statements, which had exhorted Catholics to vote against the party in power but refrained from attaching penalties for failure to do so, this last letter explicitly imposed ecclesiastical sanctions upon Catholic *populares* placing party loyalty over religious persuasion. The letter went on to explain that a vote for the PDP was sinful because it constituted "disobedience against God, disobedience against the bishops, and an act by a Catholic against his own Catholic convictions."[27]

Archbishop Davis justified this more radical stance by indicating that the church in Puerto Rico was "no longer on the defensive" concerning such issues as birth control. He also singled out "the birth controllers and the social scientists with an itch to remake a culture and a whole people" as particular culprits in the "rising tide of paganism" taking hold of Puerto Rico.[28]

Faced with this new threat, Muñoz tried to mollify the bishops and placate his constituents. The secretary of health, Dr. Guillermo Arbona, roundly denied the existence of a government-sponsored birth control program and sterilization campaign. He indicated that contraceptive services, including the church-approved rhythm method, were provided as part of a maternal and child care program and that this program fully respected the patients' religious convictions and personal preferences. Sterilization was performed solely for medical reasons, whenever a physician felt it was necessary to protect the health or life of a patient.[29] This explanation was complemented by an advertisement published by the Family Planning Association which stressed that its activities were carried out under private auspices and defended the laws enacted in 1937.[30]

Three days before the election, Muñoz broadcast a message clarifying his party's platform. The PDP program, he stated, was not in conflict with Christian morality or principles; it was based on "the two fundamental commandments on which democracy and human freedom are based: love God above all things, and love thy neighbor as thyself." Nothing in the party's platform contradicted the Ten Commandments. Nevertheless, Muñoz reiterated the PDP's position concerning the separation of church and state and its espousal of the principle of religious tolerance. "The State does not have the right to enact the laws of one church when these are contrary to those of other churches. Each believer is bound by his conscience to obey the laws of his church. But he cannot, through the power of the State, impose those laws on those who believe in other churches."³¹

This addendum to the PDP program did little to assuage the bishops. They reaffirmed their previous ban and asserted that Catholics voting for the party did so under pain of sin. Despite Muñoz's conciliatory gestures, the impasse between the church and the PDP remained.

As election day approached, the climate of uncertainty and tension increased. The CAP invoked "red-scare" tactics, using Cuba as an example. In an advertisement published the day before the elections the CAP alluded to that government's takeover of Catholic schools as a warning of what could happen in Puerto Rico.³² It was rumored that Bishop McManus, who felt personally threatened, had obtained a permit to carry a gun.³³ This earned him the nickname "Pistol-Packing McManus," contributing further to the prevailing turbulence.

Amidst this volatile situation Muñoz's confidence slackened. Although he had attracted the usual enthusiastic crowds while on the stump, he was aware that many Catholic *populares* felt torn and deeply troubled. A few had defected to the CAP or decided not to vote. For many others, the choice between their religious faith and their political allegiance posed a serious dilemma. Some claimed to be undecided, awaiting a sign or signal to guide them in their vote; others trusted the Holy Ghost to enlighten them upon entering the voting booth. In the absence of reliable polls, the outcome of the election was difficult to predict.

By the evening of the election the suspense was over. The PDP had won a resounding victory, capturing 58.3 percent of the vote. It won in all the municipalities except one, in which the SRP emerged victorious. The CAP achieved less than 7 percent of the vote, hardly enough to claim even a moral triumph. The situation was summed up by Archibald MacLeish in a poem entitled "Moral Reflections on the Infallibility of Bishops" and dedicated to Muñoz Marín. It included the following lines:

God, say the Bishops, consider it sin
To vote in the voting for Muñoz Marín. . . .

But after the vote in the voting was done
God sent the sea as before and the sun
Though Muñoz Marín had triumphantly won. . . .

The moral is something like this, and I quote:
When the Church tells the people how God means to vote
It better begin, before damning their souls,
By taking a couple of Galluping polls.³⁴

The prelates, however, were not in a mood for humor. Although Muñoz's victory speech was deliberately conciliatory and low-keyed, the church-state conflict did not subside. Embittered by their loss, some members of the clergy became vindictive and sought to take reprisals against Catholics who had voted for the winning party. The pastor of San Juan Cathedral announced that "all those that disobeyed the order of the bishops [could not] receive the sacraments until they [had] confessed."[35] Similarly, a circular letter issued by the Archdiocese of San Juan declared that the church could excommunicate those that had not followed the bishops' ban against voting for the PDP.[36]

As the bickering threatened to flare up again, both sides sought to reach a truce. The PDP tried to "clarify" its platform once more, indicating that it did not intend to undermine Christian morality.[37] Archbishop Davis finally put an end to the turmoil by declaring that the Catholic Church of Puerto Rico would not impose any penalties on those that had voted for the party.[38]

Following this settlement, the board of directors of the Family Planning Association called on Muñoz Marín to propose that birth control services be expanded under government sponsorship. With the religious opposition effectively trounced, they felt that the time was ripe for the Health Department to embark on a full-fledged family planning program. Muñoz heard them out, but broached the matter gingerly. Privately, he said, reiterating his previous statements on this subject, he favored birth control and endorsed the efforts of the FPA; publicly, he would not touch the subject "with a ten-foot pole."[39]

In the Health Department, however, subtle changes gradually strengthened the available contraceptive services. While the policy of "local option" remained in effect—thereby providing each health unit with a measure of autonomy over services dispensed—the majority offered their patients some means of contraception. In 1962 the secretary of health gave instructions to the effect that contraceptive clinics were to be identified as such rather than be included under the general rubric of gynecological services.[40] While hardly a breakthrough, this decision made public those services that had been kept under cover.

A more significant event occurred in 1963, when the secretary of health approached Dr. José Nine Curt, the medical director of the northeast health region, about the possibility of establishing a family planning program in that region. The choice of the northeast region was particularly appropriate. The regional base hospital was the teaching facility for the University of Puerto Rico School of Medicine and therefore tended to welcome innovations in the areas of research, education, and service. This region had a population of 900,000 inhabitants, approximately 40 percent of the island's total; any pilot program that was successfully tested in the northeast area could thus be extended to the rest of Puerto Rico with relative ease. Furthermore, Dr. Nine was known to be a practicing Catholic and had a good relationship with the church. As medical director he was instrumental in providing religious services within the university hospital and had hired Father Anthony Reilly, a Franciscan priest, and an Evangelical minister to serve as "psychological counsellors" to patients.

Because of the relationship that had already been established between Nine and Father Reilly, the latter was an obvious choice to discuss family planning with other representatives of the church. The priest had come to recognize the need for such services and agreed to discuss the matter with Archbishop Davis.[41]

Despite his earlier pronouncements, Davis was flattered to have been consulted and was receptive to what Reilly, acting as a spokesman for Nine, had to say. Throughout the discussions Nine stressed that he was seeking not the church's blessing but rather its adoption of a policy of noninterference. Davis was willing to grant this so long as the rhythm method was included as one of the program's offerings, health workers were not required to prescribe measures to which they objected, the program was on a voluntary basis, and contraception was not openly promoted.[42] In addition, the archbishop agreed to meet with a group of carefully selected priests and physicians to begin familiarizing them with the church-approved rhythm method of birth control.[43]

Following this preliminary accord, Nine met with the faculty of the medical school's Department of Obstetrics and Gynecology to plan the incorporation of the rhythm method into the services offered by the health centers of the northeast region. This meeting was attended by several Catholic physicians who agreed to begin providing services in one health center.

Because these understandings implied a shift in the church's position, all parties resolved to keep confidential the negotiations and the decisions reached. Nevertheless, both Archbishop Davis and Dr. Nine pledged to face the situation unflinchingly if any information reached the press. This part of the bargain was put to the test on August 7, 1963, when the *New York Times* published an article on Puerto Rico as part of a series on the subject "Catholics and Birth Control." The article gave a detailed description of the church-state concordat and the quid pro quo that it entailed:

No formal pronouncement has been made, nor will it be made out of fear that an official public declaration may jeopardize the program, but the agreement calls for the Department of Health to disseminate full information of the church approved rhythm system of birth control.

In exchange for offering a full and fair presentation of all methods of birth control, and leaving it up to each applicant to make the specific choice, the Department of Health understands that the Catholic hierarchy will cease blanket attacks against the Government's program.[44]

The information contained in the article, which was reprinted in the *San Juan Star*, did not fail to cause a stir in Puerto Rico. Questioned about the agreement with the Health Department, Archbishop Davis indicated its tentative nature but affirmed that "we are on the track of something." He also expressed confidence about reaching "an understanding leading to positive cooperation," adding that this would require "much preparation" on the part of the church.[45]

In fact, church officials proved to be more willing to cooperate than some of their followers. Apprised of the archbishop's stance, several Catholic laymen entreated him to explain his position publicly. These petitions charged that the proposed plan violated both natural law and church dogma and urged Davis to end the "grave confusion" prevailing among Catholics.[46]

Pressured by these reactions, Davis was forced to withdraw his approval of the Health Department's plan. He therefore issued a statement declaring that the Catholic church could "neither endorse nor support a plan . . . aimed at spreading contraceptive practices" and reaffirming the church's traditional stand against birth control. However, the prelate's statement recognized that the Catholic position on contraception was not held by members of other faiths and said that the church could not "force its attitude on those who do not share it."[47] This represented a marked departure from the bishops' position prior to the 1960 elections. Thus, Archbishop Davis's retraction of the agreement was interpreted as a significant step forward by the advocates of family planning, since it recognized the right of non-Catholics to make their own decisions concerning contraception. As stated by the reporter from the *New York Times*, this meant that the Catholic church and its members could "insist upon the right to *propose* their own views and *oppose* positions they hold to be wrong, but never to *impose* their own moral doctrines upon individuals who do not accept the Catholic teaching."[48]

13. Out of the Closet

By the mid-1960s Puerto Rico had begun to experience a number of economic changes. Following a relaxation of the U.S. tariff structure, Third World countries with large reserves of cheap labor began to undercut Puerto Rico's trade with the mainland and to attract the light, labor-intensive industries that Fomento had promoted over the previous two decades.[1] The island's industrial policy shifted toward attracting large petrochemical plants, which were felt to have greater stability because of their rigid locational requirements and the massive capital investment needed for their establishment. In addition, this type of heavy industry provided jobs for men and promised to produce the raw materials needed by other industries, thereby inducing other manufacturers to locate in Puerto Rico. "Vertical integration" and "downstream industries" became the magic words through which Fomento's planners hoped to revive the Bootstrap mystique.

Petrochemicals, however, provided more pollution than jobs. The limited employment opportunities that were created required specialized skills and technical know-how and were therefore unable to make an impact on Puerto Rico's high rate of unemployment. Moreover, the downstream industries failed to materialize, and the much-heralded multiplier effect on which employment projections had been based had to be drastically revised.

The island's economic situation was further exacerbated by a change in the migratory trends. The population outflow of the 1950s became a negligible stream in the 1960s; in fact, in three years (1961, 1963, and 1968) there was a net population gain through in-migration. Returning migrants, together with an influx of Cubans and Dominicans, increased the population by approximately two hundred thousand between 1960 and 1970.[2]

The growing imbalance between jobs and workers called for new social, economic, and political policies. The government, however, proved unwilling to abandon the formulas that had served it so well. Muñoz Marín's handpicked successor, Roberto Sánchez Vilella, elected in 1964, entered office promising "new ideas, new faces, a new style." Yet, despite the veneer of change, the PDP remained wedded to its earlier development strategy; Sánchez Vilella's program was simply a linear extrapolation of Muñoz's policies. Queried about his stance on birth control in 1967, the governor replied, "There's no secret about it. We haven't changed anything. It's the same policy we've had for years."[3] A similar answer would have been equally applicable with respect to many other issues.

The controversial and much-delayed family planning program in the northeast region finally got under way in January 1965; by then bishops Davis and McManus had been replaced by Puerto Ricans, and the church was vigilant but not vocal. Services in the region were provided by itinerant physicians and nurses, and a variety of medically approved contraceptive measures were offered to women in the sixteen municipalities covered by the program.

This limited effort and the activities of the Family Planning Association were strengthened as a result of federal initiatives in birth control. Contraception had gained prominence as an issue in 1959 following a report by General William H. Draper, who had been appointed by President Eisenhower to head a commission to study the foreign aid and military assistance programs of the United States. In his report, Draper stated that foreign aid, especially in Latin America, could not succeed as long as excessive population growth continued. The report therefore recommended that a portion of this aid be devoted to making the developing countries aware of the problems that accompany population growth.[4] Eisenhower did not adopt this recommendation, however. Asked in 1959 about the federal government's relation to birth control, he answered: "I cannot imagine anything more emphatically a subject that is not a proper political or governmental activity or function or responsibility. . . . That's not our business."[5]

Nevertheless, by 1965 birth control had become part of the federal government's business. In 1965, President Lyndon B. Johnson referred to the world population explosion in his state of the union address and indicated his resolve to apply knowledge to curb the rate of growth. Later the same year the president spoke of the need to "face forthrightly the multiplying problems of our multiplying population."[6] Alluding to Stephen Enke's computations and conclusions on the economic aspects of slowing population growth, Johnson urged an international audience celebrating the twentieth anniversary of the United Nations to "act on the fact that less than $5.00 invested in population control is worth $100.00 invested in economic aid."[7] Relying upon this economic rationale for the support of birth control practices, federal policy sought to promote contraception as part of its health and welfare programs.

In 1965 the Office of Economic Opportunity (OEO) became the first federal agency to offer direct grants exclusively for birth control. Because the support of the Sunnen Foundation was coming to an end, the FPA applied for an OEO grant of approximately five hundred thousand dollars to continue providing birth control services. The funds became available in mid-1966, and the association once again reactivated its program. This covered all of Puerto Rico, with the exception of the Northeast health region, and offered a wide variety of contraceptive methods: creams, jellies, foams, suppositories, condoms, diaphragms, IUDs, pills, and materials for the rhythm method.[8]

Because OEO guidelines explicitly prohibited the use of federal funds for sterilization, this procedure was not among the FPA's offerings. Nevertheless, the association found a way around this restriction. Since it had promoted surgical sterilizations for over a decade, the FPA had an effective network of providers to which it could refer patients. As requests for *la operación* continued, an ingenious referral system was devised. For example, the FPA would refer a prospective applicant to a women in Bayamón, who made arrangements to have the patient admitted to the municipal hospital of Barceloneta. The intermediary collected a fee of ten dollars for this service, and the municipal hospital received an additional seventy-five dollars for the operation. The municipality in turn hired a doctor who would perform an average of eight sterilizations every Friday. Patients admitted on Thursday would be operated on the following day and discharged on Sunday.[9] Those who could not afford to pay the full eighty-five-dollar fee were assisted by members of the FPA staff, who used their personal contacts to have laboratory tests performed free of charge in public facilities.[10] This artful combination of federal funds, free enterprise, and public services made it possible for the FPA to reach a wide clientele and provide a full array of contraceptive services. Still, the association continued to fret over the commonwealth's ambivalent attitude toward birth control and hoped for a breakthrough permitting "an open program of family planning services through the whole system of public health units and maternity hospitals of Puerto Rico."[11]

This hope began to materialize through the enactment of additional federal legislation promoting family planning. In the early 1960s, President Kennedy had made services to the mentally retarded one of his health priorities, and research in this area was generously supported. Government-sponsored studies determined that the incidence of mental retardation was associated with premature births and that prematurity was more common among young, poor women who had children in quick succession without adequate prenatal care.[12]

Responding to this finding, Congress passed the Maternal and Child Health and Mental Retardation amendments to the Social Security Act, providing funds for prenatal care. Initially, this care excluded contraception; in 1967, however, further amendments to the act specified that no less than 6 percent of funds for maternal and child health services were to be spent on family planning. As one of the beneficiaries of the federal programs, the commonwealth Health Department was obliged to comply with this requirement, and its birth control activities were accordingly strengthened. Nevertheless, the open program that the FPA advocated awaited more fundamental changes in politics and policies.

This occurred in 1968, when the long reign of the PDP came to an end. Intraparty power struggles, together with the increasing disaffection of the emergent middle class, had weakened the party's electoral strength. The New Progressive party (NPP), a thinly disguised version of the old Statehood Republic party, captured a plurality of the vote, and Luis A. Ferré became Puerto Rico's third elected governor.

As a candidate, Ferré had forcefully denounced public sponsorship of contraception and stressed his personal, Catholic conviction against birth control. Pointing out that Pope Paul VI's encyclical *Of Human Life* condemned not only contraceptive pills but also the rhythm method when used with the express purpose of avoiding conception, Ferré expressed the opinion that "no political party should proclaim that it will use the people's money . . . to carry out a program which is diametrically opposed to the official position of a church."[13] In keeping with this statement, the NPP avoided all mention of family planning or population control in its 1968 platform.

Once in office, however, the NPP leadership backed out of this categorical stance and began establishing the foundation for a significant change in policy. In January 1969 the secretary of social services named a "coordinating committee" to study Puerto Rico's population problem and to recommend a birth control policy for the island.[14] In an obvious attempt to ward off political attacks from the PDP, he designated Teodoro Moscoso committee chairman. The rest of the group included representatives of key government agencies and the news media, prominent economists and demographers, the executive director of the Family Planning Association, civic and political leaders, and a Catholic priest.

While the committee was meeting and drafting its report, its members also began to prepare a political climate that would be receptive to its recommendations. The population issue was repeatedly discussed in lectures and press conferences, newspaper articles, and television programs. Moscoso invited Ernest Gruening and members of the Ford Foundation to Puerto Rico, where they met with Governor Ferré to discuss the problems of population growth.[15] Apparently convinced by the visitors' arguments, Ferré indicated his interest in starting a family planning program under government auspices; however, he feared that the PDP opposition would attack him both for changing his mind and for adopting a policy in conflict with Catholic doctrine. Moscoso assured the governor that this type of opposition could be preempted and set out to prove it. Accompanied by Gruening and an editor from *El Mundo*, Moscoso approached Muñoz Marín concerning the proposed change in population policy. Muñoz agreed to remain silent, thereby muffling any criticism from the PDP and allowing the NPP and the study group to continue with its original plans.[16]

The committee submitted its report in October 1969. After describing the island's demographic situation and the socioeconomic implications of unabated population growth, the report concluded that the government had the "unavoidable obligation to sponsor as soon as possible the most vigorous and effective program . . . of orderly and rational family planning."[17] Marshaling a variety of data and authoritative sources, the committee justified its advocacy of birth control on eugenic, health, and economic grounds. It was argued that the quality of the population was more important than its quantity and that "small families, whose children are responsibly borne, well cared for, and educated, are those that tend to produce the quality of person and society to which we aspire."[18] The health rationale did not indicate the advantages of adequate child spacing; rather, the report provided evidence that infant mortality tends to increase with rising birth order and cited a variety of sources whose studies had shown a negative relationship between birth order and noteworthiness.[19]

It was the economic rationale, however, which dominated the committee's report. Unchecked population growth was seen as increasing unemployment, aggravating the skewed distribution of income, and imperiling social mobility. Moreover, it found poverty and high fertility inextricably related, each reinforcing the other and perpetuating the dependency of the population on government programs. Investing in birth control was therefore justified as a means of precluding future expenditures in such publicly subsidized services as housing, education, and health care. Even in the short run, the economic benefit of preventing a birth was estimated to be three times as high as its cost.[20]

The committee proposed the establishment of an island-wide family planning program aimed at reaching a target population of two hundred thousand fertile, medically indigent women.[21] Because the plan rejected sterilization as a means of contraception and was based on the voluntary participation of the clientele, it was approved by the priest serving on the committee. Because it also contemplated a role for the Department of Health, the Department of Social Services, and the Family Planning Association, it was endorsed by representatives of each of these three agencies. This broad base of support enhanced its political appeal and facilitated its adoption.

Overcoming his earlier hesitancy, Ferré incorporated the committee's recommendations into his annual state of the commonwealth message to the legislature. The new policy on birth control was officially announced on January 14, 1970. Calling overpopulation the "greatest obstacle" to Puerto Rico's continued social and economic development, the governor proposed extending to the entire island "a formal voluntary program of family planning orientation and services."[22] At least one journalist pointed out that, ironically, Puerto Rico had had to wait for a practicing Catholic to become governor before family planning was "take[n] out of the closet and [made into] an islandwide government program."[23]

Despite token protests, Ferré's proposal was favorably received.[24] In a surprise move, the Catholic episcopacy declared its willingness to assist in solving Puerto Rico's population problem as long as the "solutions are in accordance with Church doctrine."[25] Bishop Luis Aponte Martínez, acting as a spokesman for all the bishops, indicated that decisions concerning childbearing and contraception were "a responsibility of each individual before God," thereby eschewing the possibility of church intervention.[26] These statements were therefore widely interpreted as a qualified approval for a government-sponsored family planning program.[27]

Aimed at "giving each Puerto Rican mother and child a better chance to attain a healthier, fuller life," the proposed effort sought to integrate the existing programs and to reallocate responsibilities among the three main participating agencies.[28] The Health Department was responsible for the provision of all medical services, using its local facilities for this purpose. The Department of Social Services was involved primarily in the outreach and follow-up of its welfare clientele and in the preparation of a master plan for public education in family planning. The Family Planning Association assumed responsibility for training all subprofessional personnel working at the local levels and for recruiting and following up those patients who were not welfare clients.[29]

Whatever its merits on paper, the proposed division of labor did not work in practice. The Department of Social Services gave a liberal interpretation to its outreach function: it acquired vans equipped as clinics and traveled throughout the island recruiting patients and providing direct services. The Health Department objected to the creation of this parallel system, and it resented becoming dependent upon clients recruited by others. The Family Planning Association similarly resisted its reduced responsibilities; although it had always supported and lobbied for the creation of a government family planning program and anticipated evolving into a monitoring and research agency concerning population matters, it was now neither a direct provider nor an effective watchdog. Moreover, it had an ill-defined clientele to recruit and no assurance that it would be adequately cared for once it was referred to the Department of Health.

The petty jealousies between the three components of the program were further compounded by the fact that each agency had a legitimate claim to primacy. The Health Department was in charge of coordinating the entire effort, and thus sought to direct and control the outreach and follow-up functions. In addition, the service component was crucial to the program's effectiveness. The Department of Social Services, however, controlled the purse strings; it therefore exercised power through budgetary measures and was exempt from the fiscal restraints that it imposed on the others. The Family Planning Association had the longest experience in the advocacy of birth control and had amassed a creditable record in providing services; as a result, it invoked past commitment and performance in its claim to authority.

As the partnership became a tug-of-war, services inevitably deteriorated. The meshing of efforts between agencies did not take place, and patients were not recruited, served, or followed up on as the original plan had envisioned.[30] The total population reached was smaller than that anticipated, and the final outcome in births averted also fell short of the target. While the plan had projected a reduction of 9 percent in the absolute number of births, this figure actually rose between 1970 and 1972.[31] The birthrate, however, underwent a slight decrease: from 24.8 to 24.0 per 1,000 inhabitants. Despite the flourish with which it had been drafted and adopted, the family planning program had failed to attain the vigor and efficacy hoped for by its proponents.

The Ferré administration was floundering in other areas as well. Evidence of corruption among high government officials had been uncovered and widely publicized, and the polls reflected a climate of distrust among the electorate. In addition, the New Progressive party faced a reunited and reorganized Popular Democratic party under the leadership of Rafael Hernández Colón. In November 1972 the PDP was returned to power and Hernández Colón was elected governor.

With family planning no longer a politically taboo subject, the PDP expressed its support for population control in its party platform. After assuming the governorship, Hernández Colón attempted to meet this commitment by increasing the budgetary allocation for birth control and ordering the centralization of all governmental family planning programs under the direction and supervision of the Health Department.[32] This concentration of responsibility ended the interagency power struggles, but did little to reduce the strain between the government programs and the Family Planning Association. The latter felt that the department was overextending its authority by dictating to the association what its role should be and by controlling the application of its funds.[33]

Whereas the association's concerns had previously commanded little official interest, representatives of the government now sought to heal the breach between the private agency and the makers of public policy. Luis Muñoz Marín accepted an invitation to address the members of the FPA at their annual meeting; in his speech he stated that the fundamental problems confronting Puerto Rico could not be solved without first controlling population growth.[34] Moscoso, once again in charge of Fomento, also activated his interest in population control, asking General William H. Draper to send a high-level team to advise Hernández Colón on Puerto Rico's current population and family planning program.[35] Although General Draper had not been able to persuade Eisenhower to make birth control the business of government, Moscoso apparently felt that the general, now director of the Population Crisis Committee, would have greater success with the governor of Puerto Rico.

The PDP's revived interest in family planning was at least partly prompted by the island's economic plight. The GNP that had grown by 7.3 percent in fiscal 1973 almost stopped growing the next year.[36] Construction, which had boomed during the 60s, was virtually paralyzed in 1973.[37] Because the petrochemical industry had relied on Venezuelan crude oil, the manufacturing sector was severely crippled by the oil price explosion. The subsidiary plants, which had been so carefully promoted, began closing down when their "upstream" supply sources ceased production. The official rate of unemployment, which had hovered around 12 percent even in the prosperous Bootstrap years, rose ominously, reaching 19.3 percent in 1976.[38]

Although the full impact of the recession was partly cushioned by increased government spending and the doubling of federal grants-in-aid and transfer payments coming into the island, these measures exacted a political price. The economy of the island was more definitively integrated with that of the United States, and Puerto Rico's future came to be more firmly tied to the ebb and flow of circumstances external to it. As the locus of major economic decisions shifted to Washington, Venezuela, and even Iran and Saudi Arabia, the commonwealth's lack of autonomy was highlighted. This in turn seemed to enhance the relevance of birth control; in the dynamics of dependent development, population growth stood out as one of the variables over which the government could exert some influence.

Moscoso's request to General Draper was answered in December 1973, when a joint team from the Population Crisis Committee and the International Planned Parenthood Federation visited Puerto Rico. The field trip had a twofold purpose: looking into the current relationship between the government and the FPA, and advising the governor on the birth control program. As part of its first task the team met with the board of directors and staff of the FPA and found that they wanted the government to permit them to operate without external interference, while providing them with federal funds. Team members therefore promised to stress the importance of maintaining the autonomy of the FPA during their meeting with the governor, which they subsequently did.[39]

The data gathered by the visitors showed that Puerto Rico's family planning program was already extremely well financed by the federal Department of Health, Education and Welfare. Indeed, they concluded that, on a per capita basis, the program was "much more liberally funded than any other program . . . anywhere in the world."[40] At the same time, the government's efforts were falling short in delivering contraceptive services and in curbing the birthrate. The team thus concluded that the available resources had to be better utilized and aimed toward specific demographic targets.

In its meeting with the governor, the visiting team emphasized two points: "*First*, the need to treat family planning on a plane equal to maternal-child health rather than as simply a part of it. *Second*, because the issue of population is so much broader than simply providing services, cutting across the spectrum of government departments, it might be advisable to establish some sort of Cabinet-level committee to coordinate policy."[41]

Hernández Colón responded positively to the first suggestion, immediately instructing the secretary of health to establish the family planning component separate from, and parallel to, the department's maternal and child health program. The governor was less receptive to the second recommendation, indicating that he already had ninety-three committees reporting directly to him and did not want to set up any more.[42]

The government's renewed commitment to birth control was embodied in the governor's state of the commonwealth address of 1974. Referring to family planning as the "indispensable foundation in starting to find a real solution to . . . unemployment and many other basic problems besetting the country," the governor proposed the creation of an assistant secretariat for family planning within the Health Department.[43]

In February 1974, Dr. Antonio Silva Iglecia, a gynecologist in private practice, was designated assistant secretary for family planning and given responsibility for implementing a "vigorous policy of family planning on a voluntary basis." The FPA was once again charged with recruiting and following up the program's clientele.

Although the program was located within the Health Department, its major objective was population control; accordingly, Silva initially sought to achieve replacement-level fertility, or zero population growth, by 1984, a target that was subsequently considered to be unattainable.[44] Unlike the program begun under the Ferré administration, which interpreted the high incidence of female sterilization as a sign of despair, creating an obligation to offer women "less dramatic means to solve their family planning problems," the new program included a sterilization campaign as part of its efforts to reduce the birthrate.[45] Thus, in one of his first interviews, Dr. Silva noted that while he was not sure whether sterilization was good or bad, he felt that it was necessary. Pointing out that 35 percent of all Puerto Rican women in the childbearing ages had already been sterilized, he expressed the hope of increasing the number of men undergoing vasectomies to an average of one hundred per week.[46] Later, the total number of sterilizations planned for fiscal year 1974–75 was set at five thousand.[47]

Within a short time, the family planning program reached into every island town. By June 1974, scarcely four months after it began operating, the program had an active clientele of ninety-six thousand. Some fifteen sterilization centers had been established, and an equal number were being planned. A few private hospitals were contracted to provide surgical services, and these were kept busy processing program clients on an assembly-line basis. A total of 1,050 sterilizations had been performed, most of these on women.[48] Not surprisingly, although sterilization was but one component of the family planning effort, it became the most visible and controversial aspect of the program. In his zeal, Silva ran roughshod over Catholic sensitivities, feminist concerns, federal regulations, and pro-independence sympathies.

Shortly after his appointment, Silva initiated talks with Cardinal Aponte Martínez in an effort to "avoid a repeat of the 1960 state-Church birth control controversy."[49] After one of the talks, he spoke to the press to imply the cardinal's tacit approval of the family planning program. The cardinal strongly denied any such complicity, denouncing the sterilization effort and threatening to stir up further opposition to the program.[50] Hernández Colón, whose Catholic credentials were unimpeachable, was called upon to arbitrate the dispute. In a meeting with the governor, the cardinal stated that he was not against the ends of the program but that he objected to the means through which it was being carried out. He was particularly offended by the established demographic targets, which set the number of procedures to be carried out monthly in each health region.[51] Hernández Colón agreed that Silva's targets sounded like compulsory quotas and that these conflicted with the stated voluntary nature of the program.[52]

In his defense, Silva argued that the projected figures were merely the quantitative standards required for planning, evaluation, and budgeting. He also stressed that sterilization was not actively promoted but rather provided in response to patient demand.[53] Nevertheless, the physician was overruled by the governor, who vetoed the use of targets and assured the cardinal that the program would protect the freedom of conscience of both providers and beneficiaries.[54]

The feminists' complaint against the program also concerned its liberal policy on sterilization. Ironically, Silva had co-opted the feminist cry for women's control over their own bodies and ended the de facto restrictions governing *la operación*. Traditional age and parity requirements were waived as "undignified" and unnecessarily paternalistic, and all emancipated minors and persons over twenty-one years of age became eligible for sterilization.[55] The feminists, who felt that the goal of "bodily self-determination" was being subverted to the ends of population control, found themselves in the anomalous position of advocating restrictions on the performance of tubal ligations and other surgical procedures. They felt that only more restrictive guidelines could provide safeguards against the abuse of sterilization.

The Commission on Women's Rights was particularly worried about the sterilization of minors, which raised questions concerning the possibility of coercion and the abrogation of informed consent. The program's rapid expansion of sterilization services, its targeting of an indigent clientele, its mass-production techniques, and its emphasis on checking population growth reinforced the suspicion that the program entailed coercion. In a letter to the governor and Dr. Silva, the commission asked that the family planning program put an end to the sterilization of minors.[56]

The U.S. Department of Health, Education and Welfare also intervened to enforce federal norms that prohibited the sterilization of women under twenty-one. Alleging that its sterilization effort was locally funded and that commonwealth law gave married minors the legal rights and duties of an adult, the Health Department planned to challenge the imposition of federal guidelines in court.[57] Silva specifically objected to the fact that HEW, although a "minority stockholder" in the commonwealth's family planning enterprise, could dictate the operation of the program as a whole, including those services that it was not sponsoring directly.[58]

As the situation involved not only the ethics of health care and population control but also the ambivalent relationship between Puerto Rico and the United States, it was solved politically rather than judicially. In June 1976, after approximately one hundred minors had been operated on, Governor Hernández Colón ordered the family planning program to halt all sterilizations of persons under twenty-one years of age.[59] This moratorium, however, scarcely dampened the program's efforts. Between fiscal years 1974–75 and 1976–77, the Health Department sponsored over twenty-nine thousand sterilizations, 90.4 percent of these on women.[60]

Given the size, thrust, and auspices of the program, proindependence groups condemned it as genocidal. Complaints were also made that the government was welcoming an influx of foreigners at the same time that it was promoting birth control among Puerto Ricans.[61] This criticism was at least partially blunted by commonwealth efforts to curb immigration. In October 1975 an advisory group on Puerto Rico created by President Nixon and Governor Hernández Colón recommended a revised compact of permanent union between the United States and Puerto Rico. One of the powers requested by the commonwealth under the new compact was that of controlling the entrance of aliens into the island. In December 1975 the proposed compact was submitted to the U.S. Congress, where it died in committee; the commonwealth was thus caught in the paradoxical situation of lacking the political power required to obtain political power.

Despite the impetus given to contraception between 1974 and 1976, no significant decrease occurred in the birthrate. After a slight decline between 1974 and 1975, the rate stabilized at 22.6 in 1976 and 1977.[62] While the relative insensitivity of this rate to changes in the provision of birth control services could be largely explained by a rise in the proportion of women in the childbearing ages, this gave small comfort to the advocates of family planning in Puerto Rico.

In 1976, Hernández Colón was defeated by NPP candidate Carlos Romero Barceló. The mayor of San Juan during the previous eight years,

Romero had been an early and staunch supporter of birth control.[63] Under his administration services nevertheless underwent a marked change in both scope and thrust. In early 1977 the Department of Health was reorganized and the office of the assistant secretary for family planning was dismantled. Birth control was placed under the aegis of an assistant secretary for ambulatory services and integrated with other preventive and therapeutic care. The new structure, which sought to group "primary health services... in order to facilitate [their] delivery and accessibility," ended the separation of the contraceptive program and hence its saliency.[64]

The current secretary of health makes a clear distinction between family planning and population control and has opted for the former. Sterilization has been de-emphasized, and services rendered have been reduced. The number of surgical procedures performed has decreased to 40 percent of its 1976 level.[65] At the same time, abortions seem to be rising. As a result of a decision by the Puerto Rico Supreme Court in 1980, both the image and the actual practice of abortion have rapidly changed on the island. Several clinics devoted exclusively to "pregnancy terminations" are now in operation in the San Juan metropolitan area; other such proprietary ventures are starting elsewhere, and established clinics are expanding their services to include this procedure. These clinics are performing abortion on an out-patient basis. The proven safety of the vacuum aspiration technique during the first trimester of pregnancy has apparently led to a major revision in the attitude of much of the medical profession. And the female population has secured one more option for control of fertility, although it is undoubtedly a costly one for many: the going fee for the service is $150.00.

With this development, it has been estimated that as many as twenty-five thousand abortions per year are currently being performed in Puerto Rico.[66] This has reduced the number of abortions undertaken under nonmedical auspices and the tragedy involved in the medical complications associated with such abortions. No less important is the effect that this increased reliance upon abortion is likely to have on population growth. If the current estimate of twenty-five thousand abortions per year is correct, it follows that approximately one out of every four pregnancies is being terminated through this means.

This situation is comparable to that which currently prevails in the United States and throughout the world.[67] That this should be the case suggests the rapid shift in public opinion that has occurred in Puerto Rico. Yet it is significant that the Puerto Rican government has failed to make any accommodation to this change. The Health Department has successfully resisted contaminating itself with any taint of the current practice of abortion. Following the Supreme Court ruling, the secretary of health vigorously reiterated the long-standing policy of his department that abortions would be performed in public hospitals only by a committee decision that a woman was in a "life-threatening situation." The interpretation of this policy was so strict, he stated, that "only one abortion was officially performed last year in a public hospital and that was a result of a case of incest."[68]

Once again the disparity between public policy and the prevailing practice dramatically presents itself.[69] At the same time, the increasing acceptance and legitimation of abortion as a birth control measure highlight the extent of both the public and the private failure of other alternatives. In Puerto Rico as in so many countries of the world, the "population problem" continues to be the subject of emotional debate and rhetorical contention. Yet in Puerto Rico, no less than elsewhere, a public policy exists which remains to be joined with what people believe and what they in fact do.

14. Unfinished Business

The preceding chapters have summarized how a society has attempted to exercise control over its size. They have traced the multiplicity of motives that gave rise to family planning activities and the tortuous course that Puerto Rico has followed in evolving and elaborating a population policy. This has been outlined against the growing acceptance of birth control practices by the residents of the island, particularly its women. The recurrent disparity between policy and practice has been highlighted. Most often the public policy of the island has grievously lagged behind the popular aspirations and concerns of the majority of its people. Time and again, the government chose to "look the other way" and avoid explicit decisions that would have facilitated the population's access to contraception. Today there is the ever more glaring inconsistency between the increasing acceptance which abortion is coming to command among a substantial segment of the female population and its continued rejection by the government.

This account has given much emphasis to the often violent fluctuations that have marked the way most segments of the Puerto Rican population have felt about the future, manifesting confidence at one moment and profound uncertainty at the next. These cycles of hope and despair are an essential part of any explanation of the changes in birth control practice which have occurred and which will take place in the future. This sharp juxtaposing of a sense of control over their lives with the feeling of abject dependency and powerlessness is the most striking feature of this history.

These chapters have also recounted a record of events which is sometimes tragic, often discloses a substantial gap between intent and consequences, and is at best inconclusive. It is obvious that this is an unfinished history. The changes that have taken place have come through fitful starts and stops, not as the result of an even, evolutionary progression. This is the case because the subject of contraception has been so inextricably intertwined with Catholicism and colonialism.

Public discussion of and public action on family planning in Puerto Rico have always been conditioned by the doctrinal position of the church. The extent to which its teaching has influenced the practices of the members of its congregation, however, is another matter. Studies of Puerto Rican fertility undertaken after World War II show little or no difference in attitudes or practice between Catholics and non-Catholics in regard to family planning. By 1968 Catholic women between the ages of fifteen and fifty had experienced an average of 3.6 live births, the exact same number as their non-Catholic counterparts.[1] Important as the position of the Catholic church has been in this history, its real influence has been confined to the arena of public debate.

The consequences of Puerto Rico's status as a United States colony have been far more complicated and obscure. Family planning initiatives were, from the point of view of Puerto Ricans at least, often capriciously canceled by the island's Washington overlords, as in 1936 when the order was issued to terminate the government's limited start in the promotion of birth control. On the other hand, Governor Ferré's conversion to the "population cause" and Governor Hernández Colón's creation of a categorical agency within the Health Department to promote family planning occurred partly as a result of the influence that leaders of such groups as the Population Crisis Committee and the Ford Foundation were able to exert.

Once the federal government entered the business of birth control, the effect of its new policies was less subtle and more pervasive. In order to obtain its share of federal funds, the Puerto Rican government was required to comply in its public program with the guidelines established by Washington, guidelines that invariably gave little or no thought to the island's distinctive socioeconomic and cultural context.

But the impact of colonialism upon this history extends beyond the continuing necessity to meet federal requirements. The political relationship between Puerto Rico and the United States facilitated the importation of capital and ideas and the export of people. The large-scale emigration of Puerto Ricans to northern cities both deflected attention from the population issue in Puerto Rico and heightened its importance in the United States. While at its height the migratory movement acted as a safety valve to reduce population growth and decrease the number of redundant workers on the island, in recent years this movement has been in both directions, with returning migrants balancing or even exceeding those that leave.

Puerto Rico's colonial status has been important in other ways as well. This has been emphasized in the international attention it has commanded as a laboratory for social and technological innovation in contraception. The island offered not only the required "cage of ovulating females" but also a cadre of cooperating professionals and a government which promoted meliorism and looked to social engineering for the solution to its economic problems. The dependency of this society upon the United States, its most prominent feature, blighted its people with uncertainty about their cultural identity and their future, and yet effectively precluded any addressing of realistic alternative arrangements so long as the island received close to $4.7 billion per year from the federal government.[2] This dependency and the insecurity it fosters have been expressed in a variety of ways. While some indulge in slavish emulation and imitation of the United States, others reject the promotion of any contraceptive measure on the island as genocidal.

The returns of the 1980 U.S. census have disclosed a new ambiguity on the part of government officials in Puerto Rico. Claiming an underenumeration of their populations, several mayors have challenged the census totals. As long as federal funds are allocated on a per capita basis, these officials have a vested interest in keeping their population figures high. Thus, their concern with containing the "population explosion" is tempered by the additional revenue-sharing funds that each increase in population will bring to the island.

The 1980 census also revealed a total population of approximately 3,125,000. Because this was significantly smaller than the anticipated head count (estimated at 4 million),[3] the figure elicited contradictory responses: relief that the population was growing at a slower rate than projected was matched by the realization that the birthrate was actually higher than that reported in the vital statistics reports, a lower denominator yielding a higher rate. The birthrate for 1980 is 22.8 per 1,000 inhabitants, similar to or even higher than that of many Latin American countries that have not been exposed to publicly subsidized contraception.[4]

The crude birthrate, however, is an imperfect indicator of the fertility decline that has actually taken place. A more accurate measure is that of births per women in the childbearing age group. This fertility rate, as indicated in Table 14.1, has undergone a significant reduction over the last eight decades. The statistics therefore support the conclusion that a major change has occurred and, according to all indications, is continuing.

At the same time, the population will certainly continue to grow, for the momentum of population increase makes this inevitable. One recent estimate, for example, indicates that even if the fertility rate were to drop to the replacement level by 1985 (a highly unlikely occurrence), the population would not stabilize before exceeding five million in the middle of the next century.[5] Undoubtedly such continued growth will require a reassessment of population policy and current contraceptive practices. Despite the very substantial reduction of the fertility level in recent decades, in the eyes of many Puerto Rico's "population problem" remains as ominous and intractable as ever. This is in large part because of the way in which the decline in fertility has been achieved.

Sterilization has become the single most important contraceptive measure for Puerto Rican women. Indeed, this practice is estimated to account for 58 percent of the decline in the birthrate.[6] Over the past two generations, it has been shown, the proportion of women of childbearing age who have been sterilized has steadily risen. If to the approximately 35 percent of the female population of reproductive age that is today sterilized is added the presumed proportion of women who are infertile, sexually inactive, or cannot conceive because of the infertility of their sexual partner, then approximately half of Puerto Rican women are no longer exposed to the "risk of pregnancy."[7]

The world "leadership" role of Puerto Rico in adopting sterilization as a contraceptive measure has been heralded by many; Puerto Rico is widely acclaimed as leading all other countries in the availability and use of volun-

TABLE 14.1. Fertility Rate for Puerto Rico, 1900–1980

Period	Births[a]	Female Population 15–49 Years of Age[b]	Fertility Rate	Percent Change between Decades
1900–1909	49,017	255,447	191.9	—
1910–1919	56,346	296,244	190.2	− 0.9
1920–1929	63,900	350,778	182.2	− 4.2
1930–1939	73,477	423,810	173.4	− 4.8
1940–1949	90,999	484,951	187.6	+ 8.2
1950–1959	82,248	520,071	158.1	−15.7
1960–1969	77,497	600,483	129.1	−18.3
1970–1979	71,294	743,930	95.8	−25.8

Source: José L. Vázquez Calzada, *La Población de Puerto Rico y su Trayectoria Histórica* (Rio Piedras: Escuela de Salud Pública, Universidad de Puerto Rico, 1978), p. 139.
a. Annual average for the period, corrected for the underregistration of births.
b. Average population for the period.

tary sterilization, especially tubal ligation.[8] Reports from other parts of the world, however, show that the Puerto Rican reliance on sterilization is being imitated elsewhere. In Panama, for example, it has recently been estimated that 29.3 percent of all married women between the ages of fifteen and forty-four have been sterilized, most of these having undergone the operation since 1970.[9] There are indications that in Brazil, Costa Rica, El Salvador, Thailand, and Korea, female sterilization is being similarly resorted to.[10] In the United States, the rate of tubal ligation performed on women fifteen to forty-four years old increased by two and a half times between 1970 and 1975.[11] Female sterilization is thus emerging in many different cultural settings as "the wave of the future" in the age-old concern of women to win control over the biological function of motherhood.

From the point of view of economist William J. Kelly, the problem of sterilization as a contraceptive measure relates to "the length of the prospective stream of births prevented and the high initial cost of the method."[12] Other far more unsettling concerns further call into question the reliance which has been put upon this means of fertility control. As currently practiced in Puerto Rico, female sterilization holds no promise of achieving population stability, if that is established as the societal goal. Women typically undergo sterilization only after they have given birth to more children than are required to maintain the total population at a constant level.[13] A survey undertaken in 1976 has indicated that sterilized women have on the average given birth to 4.0 children, one more child than those who have not undergone an operation.[14] Furthermore, sterilization is most often not resorted to until after a woman has delivered more children than she desires.

It therefore must be recognized as a contraceptive method which, however definitive, is at the same time not used by a woman to insure the realization of what she and her family want in regard to size. It is an inaccurate method, and it denies what has traditionally been the basic thrust of the family planning movement, the optimum timing and spacing of children to assure their well-being as well as the interest of the family as a unit. Female sterilization may be a foolproof and, given prevailing medical technology, an essentially irreversible method for preventing conception, but it is not a planning method. When women rely extensively upon sterilization to control family size, they are not likely to control their reproduction with vigilance prior to being sterilized. A 1976 survey of Puerto Rican women, for example, revealed that almost half of those who had been sterilized had never made use of any contraceptive measure prior to undergoing *la operación*.[15] For such women the interval between pregnancies, and resulting children, is primarily a consequence of biological considerations rather than human intention.

There is also mounting evidence that the reliance that Puerto Rican women are today individually placing upon sterilization as the means to control their fertility will occasion increasing personal regrets. Many women who have turned to this method to prevent procreation have had second thoughts about their subsequent inability to conceive. As might be expected, this is particularly the case among those who after sterilization are divorced, widowed, or deserted.[16] The divorce rate (the number of divorces for each 100 marriages) has increased dramatically in Puerto Rico. The current divorce rate—46.1 percent—exceeds that of the United States and is one of the highest in the world.[17] This rapidly rising rate is likely to increase the number of women regretting having undergone sterilization, particularly given the prevailing culture. By being unable to have more children, Puerto Rican women unquestionably reduce their ability to attract another marriage partner.

Several additional observations can be made about the practice of sterilization in Puerto Rico. It has been resorted to primarily as a female contraceptive measure. While vasectomies have been actively promoted by both the Health Department and the Family Planning Association, only a small proportion of the male population has submitted to this procedure. For most Puerto Rican men *machismo* is sufficiently strong to maintain their traditional refusal to share responsibility for procreation.

In addition, a medical elite, both within and outside the Health Department, created the demand for female sterilization even though the number of women seeking this solution exceeded the capacity of the medical delivery system. That excess demand today no longer exists, and there are cogent reasons to believe that the percentage of women of reproductive age who are sterilized has reached its peak. As those with more schooling opt for less drastic methods, the acceptance and use of alternative family planning practices are likely to become more differentiated along class lines. The resort to female sterilization, if not consistently diffused throughout the population, was at least relied upon by all layers of the society. Today it seems to be emerging as the contraceptive measure of choice of the poor and the less educated, of those in the service labor force as opposed to those employed in white-collar or manual occupations, and of those whose husbands are engaged in agricultural or blue-collar jobs.[18]

At the same time, a substantial segment of the population remains relatively unmotivated toward the practice of family planning. This includes those women who have become completely marginal to the society, who were bypassed by the hopefulness that inspired many in previous years, and who see no prospect of upward mobility. For them many children may be a rational response to personal insecurity and lack of a sense of purpose. When their children are fathered by more than one man, they gain entry into multiple kinship systems, with the economic, psychological, and social support that this affords.[19] For others the knowledge that sterilization is readily available is very likely inhibiting their reliance on other birth control alternatives or at least reducing the vigilance of their use of contraceptive measures.

The recent emergence of abortion as a relatively safe birth control option is not only rapidly altering prevailing practice but also increasing differences between classes in the alternatives they choose. The charges incurred in the abortion clinics, as opposed to the cost-free sterilization in a public institution, are likely to reinforce attitudinal differences between the classes toward this birth control measure. In Puerto Rico as in the United States, the more affluent have been able to secure abortions in the past through trips to the Virgin Islands or gynecologists prepared to perform the procedure in some of the island's most reputable hospitals. The recent opening and wide promotion of proprietary abortion clinics have changed the prevailing family planning practice of this population by introducing vacuum aspiration as an out-patient procedure and increasing accessibility to this method. What this may mean in the long run for other family planning practices remains unclear. However, proprietary abortion clinics are unlikely to provide their clients with the knowledge and skills required to prevent unwanted pregnancies, therefore avoiding further abortions.

In a highly stratified society it should not be surprising that both the acceptance of family planning and the type of birth control measures adopted should vary significantly by class. Sterilization and abortion, as these procedures are currently made available to Puerto Rican women, seem to militate against reliance upon and the effective use of other birth control methods. The failure to secure a greater acceptance of less drastic family planning practices is not the result of a lack of knowledge on the part of Puerto Rican women about such other alternatives.[20] Rather, it appears to be related to the uneven cultural and socioeconomic development that typifies this society.

What actually is involved in reducing fertility is still imperfectly understood. Indeed, researchers at the Population Council have described the "basic determinants" of fertility as being "in considerable disarray."[21] The correlation in developing countries between a decline in fertility and the reduction of infant mortality and the increase of industrialization, urbanization, and level of educational attainment remains undisputed; further, the improvement in the status of women and the character of the distribution of income within a society, as contrasted with the income level, have come to be recognized as increasingly important. But the explanation of the decline of fertility is as elusive and uncertain as ever.[22]

An analysis of the Puerto Rican experience offers compelling support to those who contend that the reduction of the fertility level of a society occurs only as an element of a much more inclusive cultural and developmental change. While some have long been committed to such a view, others have only recently reached the conclusion that a program of family planning is no more than an instrument to quicken the pace of the demographic transition once improvements in the social and economic conditions of a population are underway.[23] Most of the programmatic activity that was undertaken in Puerto Rico to promote family planning entailed, if not a denial, at least an imperfect recognition of the necessity of this kind of larger view. Puerto Rico served as a staging area for many apostles of what has come to be characterized as the "medical model" of population control. The answer was seen in the technological fix; its guidance was to be entrusted to a combination social engineer and marketing specialist.

Some who were involved in this cause in Puerto Rico, such as Joseph Sunnen, came to see the inadequacy of such a restricted approach. However, many of the leaders of the birth control establishment and its missionaries, in Puerto Rico no less than elsewhere, retain the conviction that their goals can be pursued in the traditional manner. For those alarmed over the prospect of the population explosion in the Third World, the search continues for the optimum mechanism to control births, one that is immune to objection on any religious, cultural, or aesthetic grounds. And the vigorous purveying of available birth control measures continues with an equal sense of urgency.

At present, however, new analyses are questioning both the medical and the developmental models. The alternative views of "development as the best contraceptive" and "contraception as the best developmental tool" are both opposed by those who fail to see any causal links between population control and development. Long attacked by the left as a naive and simplistic solution to the problems of poverty and unequal distribution of wealth, birth control has more recently been condemned as meddlesome, misguided, and even counterproductive by more conservative critics.[24] The premises of Malthus and the prescriptions of the neo-Malthusians are thus once again challenged and rebutted.

For Puerto Rico the debate is academic. As in the past the population-resources issue reflects and in many ways magnifies the tensions and contradictions that are inherent in the society as it is currently constituted. Given the constraints imposed by Puerto Rico's status as an adjunct of the U.S. economy, the island's social reality includes the increasing redundancy of its people and the inability of the economy to make use of the existing labor force. While the unemployment rate is officially recorded as only slightly in excess of one-fifth of the labor force, it is widely acknowledged that at least one-third is in fact unemployed or underemployed. This rise in unemployment comes at a time when the island faces massive cutbacks and an overall curtailment of the federal funds that have propped up the economy over the last decade.

Some have characterized this development as entailing a move from crisis to chaos.[25] Officials in the federal government are intent upon reducing the drain upon the public treasury which many have come to feel Puerto Rico represents. But these officials are unable to articulate an unequivocal vision of what the future political relationship between the United States and the island should be. Puerto Ricans are themselves no closer to reaching a consensus on the status issue. Particularly given these uncertainties, the perennial "population problem" creates new anxieties, even as it is seemingly used for political advantage.

Deteriorating socioeconomic conditions appear to be triggering an increase in the net out-migration of Puerto Ricans. At the same time, the threat of a massive movement of population to the States is being used to attempt to reduce the severity of the cuts in the federal dollars that Puerto Rico today receives.[26]

This situation is eroding the island's capacity for self-reliance, a capacity that has been restricted by being tied to the vagaries of the United States economy in such a way that the impact of every economic disturbance and dislocation on the mainland is disastrously multiplied on the island. But even more important, the decisions made in such a society have tended to conform to the dictates of both internal and external interests beyond popular local control.

What is called for is the mobilization of all segments of the population both in determining and actively participating in a still undefined future. It is only through such a society that a population policy and individual acts relating to human reproduction can be made to coincide. The challenge remains to make the control of population as a societal concern consonant with the control of births as a personal matter.

The personal preferences and social aspirations of Puerto Ricans can be joined only when they cease to be acted upon and begin actively to create their own future. It is then that what is personal becomes consciously socialized and what is social is effectively personalized. Perhaps out of the current turmoil a new kind of commitment to the future will emerge and, as an integral part of that, an adaptation of and more extensive reliance upon family planning.

Notes

Chapter 1

1. P. M. Ashburn, *A History of the Medical Department of the United States Army* (Boston: Houghton Mifflin, 1929), p. 196.

2. Gordon K. Lewis, *Puerto Rico: Freedom and Power in the Caribbean* (New York: Monthly Review, 1963); and Truman R. Clark, *Puerto Rico and the United States, 1917–1933* (Pittsburgh: University of Pittsburgh Press, 1975).

3. Some gold had been obtained from Puerto Rico early in the sixteenth century, and much later a very limited quantity of copper was secured. Information on the island's resource base is available in the following source: Rafael Picó, *The Geography of Puerto Rico* (Chicago: Aldine, 1974). In recent years substantial deposits of copper ore of commercial grade have been found, but as yet no steps have been taken to exploit them. Exploration for offshore petroleum is also currently underway.

4. Luis Manuel González, "The Economic Development of Puerto Rico from 1898 to 1940" (Ph.D. diss., University of Florida, 1964), p. 62.

5. For a detailed account of Puerto Rico's demographic history consult the following: José L. Vázquez Calzada, *La Población de Puerto Rico y su Trayectoria Histórica* (Río Piedras: Escuela de Salud Pública, Universidad de Puerto Rico, 1978).

6. Ibid., p. 11.

7. González, *Economic Development*, pp. 70–79.

8. Vázquez, *La Población de Puerto Rico*, p. 23.

9. For an assessment of this influence, consult the following: Julian Steward, ed., *The People of Puerto Rico* (Urbana: University of Illinois Press, 1956).

10. Lewis, *Puerto Rico*, p. 263.

11. An exception can be noted in the existence of several Protestant churches that had been established through the intercession of Queen Victoria for the benefit of some isolated colonies of British residents.

12. Quoted by Lewis, *Puerto Rico*, p. 271.

13. Howard Stanton, "Puerto Rico's Changing Families," *Transactions of the Third World Congress of Sociology* 4 (1956): 101–7.

14. Harvey Perloff, *Puerto Rico's Economic Future: A Study in Planned Development* (Chicago: University of

Chicago Press, 1950), p. 20.

15. Subsequently the venereal ineffective rate among the American troops rose to 468 per 1,000. In 1903 the U.S. Navy, to combat this problem, denied shore leave to the crews of all visiting vessels. Herman Goodman, "The Porto Rican Experiment," *Journal of Social Hygiene* 5 (1919): 185–91 (p. 185.)

16. Vázquez, *La Población de Puerto Rico*, p. 237.

17. Bulletin no. 2, Office of the Surgeon General of the Army, 1913–14, as quoted in Ashburn, *A History of the Medical Department*.

18. Clark, *Puerto Rico and the United States*, p. 110.

19. A limited number of Puerto Ricans, it can be noted, refused to accept such citizenship. Not until a generation later did the significance of this provision of the Jones Act become fully apparent.

20. Major Garvin L. Payne, "The Vice Problem in Porto Rico," *Journal of Social Hygiene* 5 (1919): 233–42.

21. Rexford G. Tugwell, *The Art of Politics* (New York: Doubleday, 1958), pp. 78–80, 227.

22. González, *Economic Development*, p. 89.

23. Arthur D. Gayer, Paul T. Homan, and Earle K. James, *The Sugar Economy of Puerto Rico* (New York, 1938), p. 33, quoted in Clark, *Puerto Rico and the United States*, p. 110.

24. In 1923 wages for the same kind of work in tobacco factories ranged from fifty cents to four dollars a day for men, but only fifty cents to two dollars a day for women. U.S. War Department, *Report of the Governor*, 1923, p. 30, quoted in Clark, *Puerto Rico and the United States*, p. 119.

25. Sidney W. Mintz, "Cañamelar: The Subculture of a Rural Plantation Proletariat," in Steward, *People of Puerto Rico*, p. 340.

26. The contraction of the Puerto Rican economy at this time is summarized in Perloff, *Puerto Rico's Economic Future*.

27. Luis Muñoz Marín, "Puerto Rico: The American Colony," *Nation*, April 8, 1925, quoted in Thomas Aitken, *Luis Muñoz Marín: Poet in the Fortress* (New York: Signet Books, 1964), p. 81.

28. *Report of Brigadier-General George W. Davis on Civil Affairs in Puerto Rico*, Report of the War Department, 1899, vol. I, part 6, p. 790.

29. Ibid., p. 789.

30. Fred Fleagle, *Social Problems in Porto Rico* (Boston: Heath, 1917), p. 118.

Chapter 2

1. Carmelo Rosario Natal, *La Juventud de Luis Muñoz Marín* (San Juan: n.p., 1976), p. 143.

2. These publications included the *Smart Set*, the *American Mercury*, the *Nation*, and the *Baltimore Sun* in the United States.

3. In 1913, Anatole France joined Rosa Luxemburg in proposing that workers undertake a "birth strike" and stop childbearing in order to reduce the flow of manpower into the industrial and military machines. David M. Kennedy, *Birth Control in America* (New Haven: Yale University Press, 1970), p. 21. In 1937, H. L. Mencken was to propose a "sterilization bonus plan" to narrow the fertility gap between the "unfit" and "the smart and the swell."

Allan Chase, *The Legacy of Malthus* (New York: Knopf, 1977), p. 362.

4. *La Democracia*, August 21, 1922.
5. *El Mundo*, June 27, 1923.
6. *El Imparcial*, July 7, 1923.
7. *El Imparcial*, July 9, 1923.
8. *La Correspondencia*, July 13, 1923.
9. *El Imparcial*, July 24, 1923.
10. Following the establishment of American hegemony in Puerto Rico, the existing criminal code was repealed in its entirety. A criminal code based on the California statutes of 1873 was adopted in 1902. Article 268 of the enacted code read as follows: "Every person who willfully writes, composes, or publishes any notice or advertisement of any medicine, or means for producing or facilitating a miscarriage or abortion, or for the prevention of conception, or who offers his services by any notice, advertisement, or otherwise, to assist in the accomplishment of any such purpose, is guilty of a felony."
11. Marcos Huigens, Martin Berntsen, and José A. Lanauze Rolón, *El Mal de los Muchos Hijos* (Ponce: n.p., 1926), p. 1.
12. Kennedy, *Birth Control*, p. 75.
13. Huigens, Berntsen, and Lanauze, *El Mal*, p. 1.
14. Ibid., pp. 6–7.
15. *El Mundo*, November 28, 1925.
16. (San Juan) *Times*, November 30, 1925.
17. Margaret Sanger, President, American Birth League, Inc., to Dr. José A. Lanauze Rolón, March 9, 1926, included in Huigens, Berntsen, and Lanauze, *El Mal*, pp. 11–12.
18. The Holland Rantos Co. was founded in the mid-1920s by a group of Sanger's friends. The company was given that name because "Holland was the first country to make diaphragms, and Rantos . . . sounded like Ramses (another manufacturer of diaphragms)." Herbert Simonds, quoted in Madeline Gray, *Margaret Sanger* (New York: Richard Marek Publishers, 1979), p. 233.
19. James Reed, *From Private Vice to Public Virtue* (New York: Basic Books, 1978), p. 95. Lanauze's two "consultants" were not on cordial terms with each other. When Sanger had visited Amsterdam in 1915, Jacobs had dismissed her as a "mere nurse" and refused to receive her. A second physician then gave Sanger a tour of the clinic. Gray, *Margaret Sanger*, p. 102.
20. *El Día*, June 11–12, 1926.
21. *El Piloto*, July 1, 1926.
22. *El Día*, July 31, 1926.
23. *El Día*, undated (c. August), 1926.
24. *El Piloto*, August 28, 1926.
25. *El Día*, July 31, 1926.
26. *El Día*, September 26, 1926.
27. This is chapter 5 of *Woman and the New Race* (New York: Blue Ribbon Books, 1920).
28. In 1930 the Ponce contingent wrote to the members of the House of Representatives urging them to vote in favor of a bill establishing "neo-Malthusian clinics." The letter was signed by Dr. Lanauze and forty-five other persons, ten of whom are identified as physicians. M. Riera López et al. to the Honorable House of Representatives of Puerto Rico, April 4, 1930, files of the Puerto Rico Family Planning Association, San Juan.
29. Miles H. Fairbank, *The Chardón Plan and the Puerto Rico Reconstruction Administration, 1934-1954* (San Juan: The Fairbank Corporation, 1978), p. 8.

30. Thomas Mathews, *Puerto Rican Politics and the New Deal* (Gainesville: University of Florida Press, 1960), p. 4.
31. Ibid., p. 8.
32. Victor Clark, *Porto Rico and Its Problems* (Washington, D.C.: Brookings Institution, 1930), p. xxiv.
33. Ibid., p. 27.
34. Ibid., p. 32.
35. Ibid., p. 50.
36. Ibid., p. 58.
37. Ibid., p. 9.
38. Ibid., p. 13.
39. Ibid., pp. 522–24.
40. Ibid., p. 520.
41. Ibid., pp. 524–31.
42. The emigration required was so large as to be unfeasible: "It would require the transfer of 50,000 people annually to other countries for a series of years and a permanent outflow of 25,000 annually thereafter to reduce the population to a point where all who remained at home could find steady and remunerative employment." Ibid., p. 520.
43. Ibid., p. 532.
44. The Association of Sugar Producers, representing the organized sugar interests, was quick to see the Brookings report as supportive of its industry. In 1936 the association had part of the study reprinted and issued under the title of *The Sugar Problem of Porto Rico* (Washington, D.C.: Brookings Institution, 1936).
45. *Porto Rico: A Broken Pledge* (New York: Vanguard Press, 1931).
46. Ibid., p. 163.
47. Ibid., p. 165.
48. Ibid., p. 88.
49. Linda Gordon, *Woman's Body, Woman's Right* (New York: Grossman Publishers, 1976), p. 337.

50. *Birth Control Review*, May 1932, p. 157.
51. Both the English version of the letter and its translation into Spanish appeared in *El Mundo*, January 27, 1932.
52. Mathews, *Puerto Rican Politics*, p. 34.
53. Ibid.
54. *San Juan Star*, September 8, 1980. The Department of Justice ordered in May 1982 a reexamination of the documents in the Rhoads case. *San Juan Star*, May 31, 1982.
55. Inaugural Address of Governor James R. Beverley, San Juan, 1932, pp. 5, 8, quoted in Truman R. Clark, *Puerto Rico and the United States, 1917–1933* (Pittsburgh: University of Pittsburgh Press, 1975), p. 151.
56. He wrote: "I have always believed that some method of restricting the birth rate among the lower and more ignorant elements of the population is the only salvation for the Island. The tragedy of the situation is that the more intelligent classes voluntarily restrict their birth rate, while the most vicious, most ignorant and most helpless and hopeless part of the population multiplies with tremendous rapidity." Beverley to Sanger, May 25, 1933, Margaret Sanger Papers, Sophia Smith Collection, Smith College, Northampton, Massachusetts (hereafter cited as MSP).
57. Beverley pointed out the persistence of hunger and poverty at the same time that the year had seen the largest crops of sugar ever raised in the island. *Thirty-second Annual Report of the Governor of Puerto Rico*, 1932.
58. Ibid., p. 8.
59. *New York Times*, September 27,

1932, and October 7, 1932, quoted in Clark, *Puerto Rico and the United States*, pp. 151–52.

60. Quoted in Arturo Ortíz Toro, Acting Attorney General, Department of Justice of Puerto Rico, to the Honorable Executive Secretary, San Juan, Puerto Rico, September 26, 1932, MSP.

61. Ibid.

62. Violet Callendar received training in contraceptive work at one of Margaret Sanger's clinics in New York. Upon her return she visited Dr. George C. Payne, director of Public Health Units at the Puerto Rico Department of Health, to solicit aid. Dr. Payne reported on the meeting: "It was not clear whether she wanted a financial contribution or other support. I told her I had no interest in the teaching of contraceptive methods to the middle and upper classes and that I considered that much study was still necessary to find a method which would effectively meet the needs of the poor." Payne to Dr. W. A. Sawyer, May 1, 1936, "Chronological Summary of Birth Control Movement in Puerto Rico in Its Relation to the Development of Public Health Units," Rockefeller Archive Center, Pocantico Hills, North Tarrytown, New York.

63. Callendar to Sanger, November 21, 1932, MSP; and Christopher Tietze, "Human Fertility in Puerto Rico," *American Journal of Sociology* 53 (1947): 38.

64. This clinic was run by an American woman, Mrs. Ralph Bermúdez, and Dr. Manuel Guzmán Rodríguez. Editorial, *Boletín de la Asociación Médica de Puerto Rico* 29 (1937): 346.

Chapter 3

1. Arturo Morales Carrión, *Ojeada al proceso histórico de Puerto Rico* (San Juan: Editorial del Departamento de Instrucción Pública, 1956).

2. James Bourne to Governor Franklin Delano Roosevelt, November 27, 1932, Democratic National Campaign Committee Correspondence, 1928–33, United States Possessions, Franklin D. Roosevelt Library, Hyde Park (hereafter cited as FDRL).

3. Rexford G. Tugwell, *The Art of Politics* (Garden City, N.Y.: Doubleday, 1958), p. 78.

4. Ibid.

5. "Inaugural Address of Honorable Robert H. Gore," July 1, 1933, quoted in *El Mundo*, July 2, 1933.

6. *El Mundo*, July 19, 1933.

7. Thomas Mathews, *Puerto Rican Politics and the New Deal* (Gainesville: University of Florida Press, 1960), p. 101 (n. 167).

8. Ibid., p. 122.

9. Ibid., p. 127.

10. Governor Gore to Johnstone, October 2, 1933, Bureau of Insular Affairs file #28659, National Archives Building, Washington, D.C. (hereafter cited as NA).

11. James Bourne, "A Constructive Plan for Puerto Rico," 1933, pp. 7–8, quoted in Kent C. Earnhardt, "Development Planning and Population Policy in Puerto Rico, 1898–2075: From Historical Evolution to a Plan for Population Stabilization," processed (Río Piedras: Graduate School of Planning, University of Puerto Rico, May 1977), pp. 22–23.

12. James Bourne to Harry Hopkins, April 18, 1934, Records of the Federal

Emergency Relief Administration, files 1934, RG 69, NA.

13. "Informe Sintético del Trabajo Realizado por la División de Actividades Educativas, Año 1934–35" (San Juan: Administración de Auxilio de Emergencia de Puerto Rico, 1935), p. 13.

14. "Social Work," article dealing with functions of PRERA sent by Franklin D. Roosevelt to Ernest Gruening, March 9, 1936, official files 400, box 49, FDRL.

15. *First Annual Report of the Puerto Rican Emergency Relief Administration* (San Juan: Bureau of Supplies, Printing and Transportation, 1935), p. 7.

16. Rexford G. Tugwell to Henry Wallace, March 16, 1934, quoted in Mathews, *Puerto Rican Politics*, p. 159.

17. "Report on American Tropical Policy with Special Reference to Puerto Rico and the Virgin Islands," submitted to the president by the Hon. R. G. Tugwell, assistant secretary of agriculture, n.d. (c. March–April 1934), p. 10, official files 400, box 47, FDRL.

18. Ibid.

19. Ibid., p. 11.

20. Fred Bartlett's File, "Memorandum for Dr. Tugwell on Puerto Rico and the Virgin Islands tour of inspection," April 2, 1934, quoted in Mathews, *Puerto Rican Politics*, pp. 162–63.

21. Ibid.

22. "Report on American Tropical Policy," p. 12.

23. Mathews, *Puerto Rican Politics*, p. 163.

24. Rafael Fernández García, personal interview, February 2, 1979.

25. "Report of the Puerto Rico Policy Commission (Chardón Report)," June 14, 1934, p. 1.

26. Ibid.

27. Ibid.

28. Ibid., pp. 6–7.

29. Ibid., p. 11.

30. Mathews, *Puerto Rican Politics*, p. 174.

31. Ibid., pp. 176, 202.

32. Ibid., p. 173.

33. Ernest Gruening, *Many Battles* (New York: Liveright, 1973), pp. 186–87.

34. Ibid., p. 28.

35. Ibid., p. 105.

36. Ibid., pp. 105–6.

37. Excerpts of Senate Concurrent Resolution Number 1, approved by the Senate and the House of Representatives on March 15, 1935, appendix C in Frederick C. Bartlett and Brandon Howell, "The Population Problem in Puerto Rico," Technical Paper Number 2, Puerto Rico Planning, Urbanizing, and Zoning Board (San Juan: Government of Puerto Rico, 1946).

38. Mathews, *Puerto Rican Politics*, p. 221.

39. James Bourne to Fellows, March 29, 1935, FERA #400, box 259, NA.

40. John J. Burke to President Franklin D. Roosevelt, February 5, 1936, official files 400, box 47, FDRL.

41. Ibid.

42. Quoted in letter from Mariana L. C. de Valdés, State Regent of the Catholic Daughters of America in Puerto Rico, to Ernest Gruening, June 5, 1935, files of the Division of Territories and Insular Possessions, Department of the Interior, file 9-8-116, box 1137, "Population-Birth Control," RG 126, NA.

43. Miguel Pou to President Franklin D. Roosevelt, June 3, 1935, NA.
44. Reverend Edwin V. Byrne to Ernest Gruening, June 3, 1935, NA.
45. Ernest Gruening to Reverend Edwin V. Byrne, July 3, 1935, NA.
46. Mariana L. C. de Valdés to Ernest Gruening, June 5, 1935, NA.
47. José Belaval, "Report," n.d. (c. 1937), Clarence J. Gamble Papers, Countway Library, Boston (hereafter cited as CGP).
48. Ibid.
49. "The Church and Reconstruction in Puerto Rico," sent by Franklin D. Roosevelt to Ernest Gruening, March 9, 1936, official files 400, box 49, FDRL.
50. Ibid., p. 32.
51. Ibid., p. 33.
52. Ibid., p. 34.
53. Ibid., p. 31.
54. Ibid., p. 26.
55. Edna Lonigan, "Population Control," September 3, 1935, p. 5, NA.
56. Ibid., p. 9.
57. Ibid., p. 10.
58. Ibid., pp. 2–3.
59. Resolution of the Scientific Session of the Annual Meeting of 1935 of the Medical Association of Puerto Rico, n.d. (c. September 1935), NA.
60. José Belaval, "Report," n.d. (c. 1937), CGP.
61. "Social Work," March 9, 1936, FDRL.
62. Madeline Gray, *Margaret Sanger* (New York: Richard Marek Publishers, 1979), p. 318.
63. José Belaval, "Report," n.d. (c. 1937), CGP.
64. Ibid.
65. Ibid.
66. Gruening, *Many Battles*, p. 200.
67. Ibid., pp. 200–201.
68. Ibid., p. 201.
69. Ibid.
70. Ibid.
71. José Belaval, "Report," n.d. (c. 1937), CGP.
72. Ibid.

Chapter 4

1. Gladys Gaylord to Clarence J. Gamble, October 26, 1936, Clarence J. Gamble Papers, Countway Library, Boston (hereafter cited as CGP).
2. Clarence J. Gamble to José S. Belaval, October 29, 1936, CGP.
3. José Belaval, "Report," n.d. (c. 1937); and José S. Belaval to Eric M. Mastner, October 31, 1936, CGP.
4. Phyllis Page, notes on conference with Ernest Gruening, Washington, D.C., October 26, 1936, CGP.
5. Ibid.
6. Phyllis Page, notes on interview with Mrs. James R. Bourne, New York, November 5, 1936, CGP.
7. Doone and Greer Williams, *Every Child a Wanted Child* (Boston: Harvard University Press for Countway Library, 1978), p. 167.
8. Phyllis Page to Clarence J. Gamble, November 23, 1936 (dated incorrectly as November 3), CGP.
9. Williams, *Every Child a Wanted Child*, p. 168.
10. Gladys Gaylord to Clarence J. Gamble, October 26, 1936, CGP.
11. José Belaval, M.D., Charis Gould, M.D., and Clarence J. Gamble, M.D., "The Effectiveness of Contraceptive Advice among the Under-

privileged of Puerto Rico," *Journal of Contraception* 3 (1938): 224.

12. Ibid., p. 225.

13. Clarence J. Gamble to H. L. Daiell, October 15, 1937, CGP.

14. H. L. Daiell to Clarence J. Gamble, December 29, 1937, CGP.

15. Phyllis Page to Rosa A. González, February 23, 1937, and Rosa A. González to Clarence J. Gamble, March 30, 1938, CGP.

16. Phyllis Page to Rosa A. González, February 23, 1937, CGP.

17. Belaval, Gould, and Gamble, "The Effectiveness of Contraceptive Advice," p. 224.

18. Phyllis Page to Carmen R. de Alvarado, April 14, 1937, CGP.

19. Clarence J. Gamble to Gladys Gaylord, March 7, 1938, CGP.

20. José Belaval, "Report," n.d. (c. 1937), CGP.

21. Clarence J. Gamble to Mrs. Carlos Torres, December 18, 1937, CGP.

22. E. Garrido Morales to Ernest Gruening, February 1, 1939, files of the Division of Territories and Insular Possessions, Department of the Interior, file 9-8-116, box 1137, "Population-Birth Control," RG 126, National Archives Building, Washington, D.C. (references from this same file hereafter cited as NA).

23. "Notas sobre el movimiento para la planificación de la familia en Puerto Rico," n.d. (c. 1960), Puerto Rico Family Planning Association Files, San Juan, Puerto Rico.

24. Monsignor Edwin V. Byrne to Governor Blanton Winship, April 2, 1937, included with letter from Michael Ready, General Secretary, National Catholic Welfare Conference, to President Franklin D. Roosevelt, April 12, 1937, official file 200, Puerto Rico, Franklin D. Roosevelt Library, Hyde Park.

25. Ready to Roosevelt, ibid.

26. Mariana L. C. de Valdés, State Regent, Catholic Daughters of America, to Hon. Franklin D. Roosevelt, April 26, 1937, NA.

27. Estella A. Torres to Mrs. Richmond Page, April 7, 1937, CGP.

28. Clarence J. Gamble to Margaret Sanger, April 12, 1937, CGP.

29. Phyllis Page to Carmen R. de Alvarado, April 14, 1937, CGP.

30. Ernest Gruening, *Many Battles* (New York: Liveright, 1973), p. 102.

31. Ibid.

32. Translation of statement issued by Rafael Menéndez Ramos, acting governor, at the time he signed the "birth control bill," May 1937, NA.

33. Ibid.

34. Williams, *Every Child a Wanted Child*, p. 170.

35. E. Garrido Morales to Ernest Gruening, May 4, 1938, NA.

36. Ibid.

37. Ironically, by arguing against contraception, these public health physicians were favoring the continuation of the high fetal wastage brought about by uncontrolled pregnancies.

38. Section of the report on Puerto Rico by Drs. Pierce and Williams of the U.S. Public Health Service enclosed in a letter from Margaret Sanger to Ernest Gruening, November 17, 1938, NA.

39. Ibid.

40. Ibid.

41. "Legal Situation of Contraception in Puerto Rico, as described by Mrs. Carlos Torres, President of the Asociación pro Salud Maternal e Infantil de Puerto Rico," June 1938, CGP.

42. Ibid.
43. Carmen R. de Alvarado to Clarence J. Gamble, November 18, 1938, CGP.
44. James Reed, *From Private Vice to Public Virtue* (New York: Basic Books, 1978), p. 121.
45. Alexander Lindley to Ernest Gruening, December 6, 1938, NA.
46. Ibid.
47. Estella A. Torres to Clarence J. Gamble, November 30, 1938, CGP.
48. Ibid.
49. Clarence J. Gamble to Carmen R. de Alvarado, December 12, 1938, CGP.
50. *New York Herald Tribune*, December 17, 1938.
51. Carmen R. de Alvarado to Clarence J. Gamble, n.d. (December 21, 1938), CGP.
52. *United States of America* vs. *José S. Belaval et al.*, no. 4589 cr., January 19, 1939.
53. Ibid.
54. Gladys Gaylord to Clarence J. Gamble, October 26, 1936, CGP.
55. Carmen R. de Alvarado and Christopher Tietze, "Birth Control in Puerto Rico," *Human Fertility* 12 (1947): 17.
56. Christopher Tietze, "Human Fertility in Puerto Rico," *American Journal of Sociology* 53 (1947): 39.

Chapter 5

1. E. Garrido Morales to Ernest Gruening, February 1, 1939, files of the Division of Territories and Insular Possessions, Department of the Interior, file 9-8-116, box 1137, "Population-Birth Control," RG 126, National Archives Building, Washington, D.C. (references from this same file hereafter cited as NA).
2. Draft of memorandum by Guillermo Arbona, n.d. (c. April 1963), Nine Curt Files.
3. George C. Payne, "Birth Control Activities in Puerto Rico," December 12, 1947, Rockefeller Archive Center, Pocantico Hills, North Tarrytown, New York.
4. José S. Belaval, "Reasons for the Decline of Mortality from Puerperal Causes in Puerto Rico during the Decade 1933–1943," *Puerto Rico Journal of Public Health and Tropical Medicine* 20 (1945): 515.
5. Part of the incentive for the midwives to attend these sessions was the replenishment of the medical supplies they carried in a black doctor's bag furnished by the Health Department. In addition, the rules and regulations governing the practice of midwifery decreed that failure to attend a training session for three consecutive months automatically resulted in the cancellation of the license.
6. Harold L. Ickes to Oswald Garrison Villard, March 30, 1939, NA.
7. José S. Belaval to Ernest Gruening, February 7, 1939, NA.
8. Carmen R. de Alvarado and Christopher Tietze, "Birth Control in Puerto Rico," *Human Fertility* 12 (1947): 17.
9. Department of Health, *Report of the Commissioner of Health to the Hon. Governor of Puerto Rico for the Fiscal Year 1939–40* (San Juan: Bureau of Supplies, Printing, and Transportation, 1941), p. 1.
10. George Martin, *Madame Secretary: Frances Perkins* (Boston: Houghton

Mifflin, 1976), p. 392.

11. José S. Belaval to Ernest Gruening, February 7, 1939, and Harold L. Ickes to Oswald Garrison Villard, March 30, 1939, NA.

12. José L. Vázquez Calzada, *La Población de Puerto Rico y Su Trayectoria Histórica* (Río Piedras: Escuela de Salud Pública, Universidad de Puerto Rico, 1978), p. 114.

13. Harvey S. Perloff, *Puerto Rico's Economic Future: A Study in Planned Development* (Chicago: University of Chicago Press, 1950), p. 33.

14. Ibid., p. 35.

15. Erich W. Zimmerman, "Staff Report to the Interdepartmental Commission on Puerto Rico" (Washington, D.C., September 9, 1940), p. 13.

16. Ibid., p. 21.

17. Charles T. Goodsell, *Administration of a Revolution* (Cambridge: Harvard University Press, 1965), pp. 10–11.

18. Thomas Aiken, Jr., *Luis Muñoz Marín: Poet in the Fortress* (New York: Signet Books, 1964), p. 132.

19. Goodsell, *Administration of a Revolution*, pp. 12–13.

20. Robert W. Anderson, *Party Politics in Puerto Rico* (Stanford: Stanford University Press, 1965), p. 71.

21. Goodsell, *Administration of a Revolution*, p. 14.

22. Ibid., p. 15.

23. Ibid., p. 19.

24. Bernard Sternsher, *Rexford Tugwell and the New Deal* (New Brunswick: Rutgers University Press, 1964), p. 322.

25. Goodsell, *Administration of a Revolution*, p. 44.

26. Sternsher, *Rexford Tugwell*, p. 298.

27. Ibid., pp. 243, 255.

28. Goodsell, *Administration of a Revolution*, p. 17.

29. *Time*, May 2, 1949, p. 34.

30. Sternsher, *Rexford Tugwell*, p. 351.

31. *Time*, May 2, 1949, p. 36.

32. Goodsell, *Administration of a Revolution*, p. 21.

33. "Message of R. G. Tugwell, Governor of Puerto Rico, to the Fifteenth Legislature at its Second Regular Session, February 10, 1942" (San Juan: Bureau of Supplies, Printing, and Transportation, 1942), pp. 11–12.

34. Goodsell, *Administration of a Revolution*, p. 22.

35. "Message of R. G. Tugwell," p. 34.

36. Rexford Guy Tugwell, *The Stricken Land: The Story of Puerto Rico* (Garden City, N.Y.: Doubleday, 1947), p. 259.

37. Rexford Tugwell, "The Place of Planning in Society," in Salvador M. Padilla, ed., *Tugwell's Thoughts on Planning* (Río Piedras: University of Puerto Rico Press, 1975), pp. 61–72.

38. Tugwell, *The Stricken Land*, pp. 261–2.

39. "Message of R. G. Tugwell," pp. 26–27.

40. Goodsell, *Administration of a Revolution*, pp. 176–77.

41. "Inaugural," *Puerto Rican Public Papers of R. G. Tugwell, Governor* (San Juan: Printing Division, Service Office of the Government of Puerto Rico, 1945), p. 7.

42. Ibid., pp. 7–8.

43. Tugwell, *The Stricken Land*, p. 36.

44. Ibid., p. 35.

45. Ibid., p. 30.

46. Ibid., p. 298.

47. Sternsher, *Rexford Tugwell*, p. 97.
48. *El Mundo*, May 7, 1937.
49. *El Mundo*, July 22, 1946.
50. José Janer, personal interview, August 29, 1978.
51. Christopher Tietze, report #17, October 7, 1947, Clarence J. Gamble Papers, Countway Library, Boston.
52. Christopher Tietze, "Human Fertility in Puerto Rico," *American Journal of Sociology* 53 (1947): 39.
53. Frederick P. Bartlett and Brandon Howell, "Puerto Rico y Su Problema Poblacional," informe técnico #2, Junta de Planificación, Urbanización y Zonificación (San Juan: División de Imprenta, Administración General de Suministros, 1946).
54. David M. Kennedy, *Birth Control in America* (New Haven: Yale University Press, 1970), p. 263.
55. Ibid., p. 262.
56. Ibid., p. 266.
57. Department of Health, *Report of the Commissioner of Health for Fiscal Year 1942–43* (San Juan: Printing Division, Office of the Government of Puerto Rico, 1944), p. 40.

Chapter 6

1. Rexford G. Tugwell, *The Stricken Land: The Story of Puerto Rico* (Garden City, N.Y.: Doubleday, 1947), p. 263.
2. Charles T. Goodsell, *Administration of a Revolution* (Cambridge: Harvard University Press, 1965), pp. 77–78.
3. Rexford G. Tugwell, *The Art of Politics* (Garden City, N.Y.: Doubleday, 1958), p. 55.
4. William C. Baggs, "Puerto Rico: Showcase of Development," *1962 Britannica Book of the Year* (Encyclopaedia Britannica, Inc.), p. 26.
5. David F. Ross, *The Long Uphill Path: A Historical Study of Puerto Rico's Program of Economic Development* (San Juan: Edil, 1969), pp. 64–73.
6. Thomas Hibben and Rafael Picó, "Industrial Development of Puerto Rico and the Virgin Islands of the United States," report of the United States Section, Caribbean Commission, July 1948, p. 151.
7. Ross, *The Long Uphill Path*, p. 75.
8. Hibben and Picó, "Industrial Development," p. 46.
9. In 1948, Moscoso announced that the government was going to sell its subsidiaries to private enterprise. Robert W. Anderson, *Party Politics in Puerto Rico* (Stanford: Stanford University Press, 1965), p. 71.
10. Teodoro Moscoso, "Industrial Development in Puerto Rico," *Annals of the American Academy of Political and Social Science* 285 (1953): 61–62.
11. Federal aid to Puerto Rico had increased from less than $3 million in 1933 to $43 million in 1942. *El Mundo*, February 7, 1946.
12. *El Mundo*, February 7, 1946.
13. *El Mundo*, February 8, 1946.
14. *El Mundo*, February 10, 1946.
15. Ibid.
16. Rexford G. Tugwell, *The Stricken Land*, p. 495.
17. Ibid., p. 592.
18. *El Mundo*, June 28, 1946.
19. Thomas Aiken, Jr., *Luis Muñoz Marín: Poet in the Fortress* (New York: Signet Books, 1964), p. 179.
20. Luis Muñoz Marín, "Introducción," *El Problema Poblacional de Puerto Rico*, Síntesis del Foro Público celebrado por la Asociación de Salud Púb-

lica de Puerto Rico en la Escuela de Medicina Tropical (San Juan: Administración General de Suministros, 1946), p. 34.

21. Manuel A. Pérez to the Honorable Governor of Puerto Rico, September 20, 1945, files of the Division of Territories and Island Possessions, Department of the Interior, file 9-8-116, box 1138, "Population, Emigration-General," RG 126, National Archives Building, Washington, D.C. (references from this same file hereafter cited as NA).

22. *Time*, May 2, 1949, p. 36.

23. Nathan Glazer and Daniel Patrick Moynihan, *Beyond the Melting Pot* (Cambridge: MIT Press, 1963), p. 93.

24. Henry A. Hirshberg, "Emigration from Puerto Rico," September 16, 1944, accompanying letter from B. W. Thoron, director, Division of Territories and Island Possessions, Department of the Interior, to Persio C. Franco, December 1, 1944, NA.

25. Ibid.

26. Ibid.

27. Quoted in ibid.

28. A. J. Jaffe, ed., *Puerto Rican Population of New York City* (New York, 1954), pp. 4, 6, cited in Oscar Handlin, *The Newcomers: Negroes and Puerto Ricans in a Changing Metropolis* (Garden City, N.Y.: Anchor Books, Doubleday, 1962), p. 142.

29. Clarence Senior, "The Puerto Rican Migrant in St. Croix," mimeographed (Río Piedras: Social Science Research Center, University of Puerto Rico, 1947).

30. Glazer and Moynihan, *Beyond the Melting Pot*, p. 98.

31. Clarence Senior, "Puerto Rican Emigration," mimeographed (Río Piedras: Social Science Research Center, University of Puerto Rico, 1947).

32. Hibben and Picó, "Industrial Development," p. 107.

33. Ibid.

34. Rafael L. Trujillo to Franklin D. Roosevelt, February 3, 1936, NA.

35. James W. Cantenbien, "Memorandum on Possible Increased Immigration of Puerto Ricans into the Dominican Republic," April 10, 1936, NA.

36. H. F. Arthur Shoenfeld to the Secretary of State, April 10, 1936, NA.

37. Cordell Hull to Harold L. Ickes, August 27, 1936, NA.

38. Ibid.

39. Tugwell, *The Stricken Land*, p. 664.

40. R. G. Tugwell to Mason Barr, November 7, 1945, NA.

41. Memorandum from Mason Barr to Director Arnold, June 12, 1946, NA.

42. Raymond E. Crist, "Reconnaissance Survey of the Possibilities of Immigration into the Dominican Republic," 1945, p. 3, NA.

43. Department of State, Memorandum of Conversation on Representative Somers Suggestions with regard to Puerto Rican Immigration to Dominican Republic, and Trade Preferences to Dominican Foodstuffs Entering Puerto Rico, May 13, 1947, NA.

44. Harry Truman to Dean Acheson, April 3, 1947, NA.

45. Memorandum from Dean Acheson to the President, May 7, 1947, NA.

46. Memorandum from Clarence Senior to D. J. O'Connor, March 20, 1947, NA.

47. Department of State, Memorandum of Conversation on Representative

Somers Suggestions, May 13, 1947, NA.
48. Ibid.
49. Department of State, Memorandum of Conversation on Puerto Rican Resettlement in Dominican Republic, August 13, 1947, NA.
50. Minutes, Emigration Advisory Committee, August 23, 1947, NA.
51. *New York Times*, August 7, 1947.
52. Minutes, Emigration Advisory Committee, August 23, 1947, NA.
53. Minutes, Emigration Advisory Committee, September 11, 1947, NA.
54. Ibid.
55. Rafael Fernández García, personal interview, February 2, 1979.
56. Teodoro Moscoso, personal interview, August 23, 1978.
57. Senior, "Puerto Rican Emigration," pp. 107–8.
58. Teodoro Moscoso, personal interview, August 23, 1978.
59. *Time*, May 2, 1949, p. 36.
60. Ibid.

Chapter 7

1. Werner Baer, *The Puerto Rican Economy and United States Economic Fluctuations* (Río Piedras: Social Science Research Center, University of Puerto Rico, n.d. [c. 1959]), pp. 27, 42, 57.
2. Harvey Perloff, "Transforming the Economy," *Annals of the American Academy of Political and Social Science* 285 (1953): 54.
3. *San Juan Star*, January 8, 1976.
4. David F. Ross, *The Long Uphill Path: A Historical Study of Puerto Rico's Program of Economic Development* (San Juan: Edil, 1969), pp. 101–2.
5. Alvin Mayne and Evelyn Ramos, "Planning for Social and Economic Development in Puerto Rico," processed (San Juan: Puerto Rico Planning Board, May 1959), pp. 17–18.
6. Jaime Ariza-Macías, Hilda Díaz de Collazo, and Elizabeth Sánchez, "Food Balance Sheet: Puerto Rico, 1967–68," *Ecology of Food and Nutrition* 2 (1973): 173–80.
7. Departamento de Salud, *Informe Anual de Estadísticas Vitales, 1977* (Oficina de Estadísticas, Análisis y Control de Información, 1978), p. 1.
8. Ibid., p. 105.
9. Conrad Seipp, "Puerto Rico: A Social Laboratory," *Lancet* 284 (June 22, 1963): 1365.
10. Departamento de Salud, *Informe Anual de Estadísticas Vitales, 1977*, p. 1.
11. In 1947 Puerto Rico's rate of natural increase reached the all-time high of 31.4 per thousand. This was considered to be "probably the highest in the world" for that year. Kingsley Davis, "Puerto Rico's Population Problem: Research and Policy," *Milbank Memorial Fund Quarterly* 26 (1948): 301.
12. José L. Vázquez Calzada, *La Población de Puerto Rico y su Trayectoria Histórica* (Río Piedras: Escuela de Salud Pública, Universidad de Puerto Rico, 1978), pp. 277, 284.
13. Ibid., p. 12.
14. Stanley L. Friedlander, *Labor Migration and Economic Growth: A Case Study of Puerto Rico* (Cambridge: MIT Press, 1965), pp. 72, 104–5.
15. There was long-standing concern about this situation. In fact, in her article "Women in Development," June Nash reports that "in Puerto Rico in the nineteen-thirties and forties the unions succeeded in getting the government to

offer special incentives to companies that gave at least two-thirds of their jobs to men." Quoted in Richard J. Barnet, "The World's Resources, Part III," *New Yorker*, April 7, 1980, p. 68.

16. Even in 1946–47, 50 percent of all families received only 18 percent of the island's total income. On the other end of the scale, 16 percent of the wealthiest families accounted for half of the income. Harvey S. Perloff, *Puerto Rico's Economic Future: A Study in Planned Development* (Chicago: University of Chicago Press, 1950).

17. Nathan Glazer and Daniel Patrick Moynihan, *Beyond the Melting Pot* (Cambridge: MIT Press, 1964), pp. 99–100.

18. "The Americas' Contribution to Public Health," address to the Annual Meeting of the Puerto Rico Public Health Association, San Juan, Puerto Rico, February 10, 1948.

19. Millard Hansen, "Training and Research in Puerto Rico," *Annals of the American Academy of Political and Social Science* 285 (1953): 111.

20. Operation Bootstrap was also claimed as demonstrating "important lessons for the mainland, and for the world," in other spheres as well. Thus Stuart Chase characterized the island as "a laboratory for racial agreement and reform." *"Operation Bootstrap" in Puerto Rico* (Washington, D.C.: National Planning Association, 1951), p. 64.

21. The appearance of change should not be confused with the reality of change. On the basis of a careful analysis of the intent of the U.S. Congress in approving the new status, a member of the law faculty of the University of Puerto Rico concluded that "though the formal title has been changed, in constitutional theory Puerto Rico remains a territory." Committee on Interim and Insular Affairs, House of Representatives, 86th Congress, 1st Session, committee print no. 15, Robert J. Hunter, *Puerto Rico: A Survey of Historical, Economic, and Political Affairs* (Washington, D.C.: U.S. Government Printing Office, 1959), p. 22.

22. Gordon K. Lewis, *Notes on the Puerto Rican Revolution* (New York: Monthly Review Press, 1975), p. 14.

23. It was in fact not even a new solution to the problem. In 1922 the Union party had proposed that Puerto Rico be incorporated into the American union as an "associated free state." And the U.S. Congress had subsequently considered, but had not enacted, such a change in status. Thirty years later, however, this was forgotten.

24. Luis Muñoz Marín, "Remarks at Harvard University on Commencement Day" (mimeographed, June 16, 1955).

25. *San Juan Star*, February 14, 1979.

Chapter 8

1. The introduction to a collection of essays describing developments in Puerto Rico between 1940 and 1952 thus made reference to a "tidal wave of humanity beating ever more destructively against the economic foundations of the island." Millard Hansen and Henry Wells, "Foreword," *Annals of the American Academy of Political and Social Science* 285 (1953): vii.

2. Harvey Perloff, "Transforming the Economy," *Annals of the American*

Academy of Political and Social Science 285 (1953): 53.

3. Quoted in Harvey S. Perloff, *Puerto Rico's Economic Future: A Study in Planned Development* (Chicago: University of Chicago Press, 1950), p. 225.

4. Department of Health, *Annual Report of the Commissioner of Health to the Honorable Governor of Puerto Rico for the Fiscal Year 1946–47* (San Juan: Printing Division, General Supplies Administration, 1948), p. 189.

5. José L. Janer, "Population Growth in Puerto Rico and Its Relation to Time Changes in Vital Statistics," *Human Biology* 17 (1945): 282.

6. Clarence J. Gamble to José S. Belaval, July 30, 1946, and José A. Belaval to Clarence J. Gamble, August 21, 1946, Clarence J. Gamble Papers, Countway Library, Boston (hereafter cited as CGP).

7. Christopher Tietze, report #19, October 9, 1946, CGP.

8. José Gándara, President, Asociación de Estudios Poblacionales, to Clarence J. Gamble, May 18, 1948, CGP.

9. Rexford Guy Tugwell, "Problems of Reconstruction in Puerto Rico," *Milbank Memorial Fund Quarterly* 26 (1948): 315.

10. C. Wright Mills, Clarence Senior, and Rose R. Goldsen, *The Puerto Rican Journey: New York's Newest Migrants* (New York: Harper and Brothers, 1950).

11. Committee on Puerto Ricans in New York City, *Report* (New York: Welfare Council of New York, 1948).

12. "Research on Puerto Rican Migration," *Newsletter of the Institute of Ethnic Affairs* 3 (March 1948), p. 5.

13. San Juan: Imprenta Venezuela, 1951.

14. Princeton: Princeton University Press, 1952.

15. Millard Hansen, "A Sociological Field Study of Fertility in Puerto Rico," Proceedings of the World Population Conference, Rome, Italy, August 31–September 10, 1954.

16. New York: Columbia University Press, 1958.

17. *The Family and Population Control: A Puerto Rican Experiment in Social Change* (Chapel Hill: University of North Carolina Press, 1959).

18. Ibid., p. 327.

19. Ibid.

20. Ibid., p. 335.

21. Ibid., p. 370.

22. Christopher Tietze to the National Committee on Maternal Health, October 20, 1946, CGP.

23. Clarence J. Gamble to José S. Belaval, July 30, 1946, CGP.

24. Christopher Tietze, "An Outline for an Experiment in Population Control," National Committee on Maternal Health, October 10, 1946, pp. 1–2, CGP.

25. Christopher Tietze, reports #1–19, September 17–October 9, 1946, CGP.

26. A. M. Marchand, Acting Commissioner of Health, to Christopher Tietze, October 16, 1946, CGP.

27. Jaime Benítez, Chancellor, University of Puerto Rico, to Christopher Tietze, October 21, 1946, CGP.

28. Christopher Tietze, report #13, October 2, 1946, CGP.

29. Christopher Tietze, report #19, October 9, 1946, CGP.

30. Ibid.

31. Christopher Tietze to the National Committee on Maternal Health, October 20, 1946, p. 3, CGP.

32. Ibid.
33. Clarence J. Gamble to Dr. Howard Taylor, Jr., Chairman, Executive Committee, National Committee on Maternal Health, October 1946, CGP.
34. Christopher Tietze to Carmen R. de Alvarado, March 3, 1947, CGP.
35. Christopher Tietze to Clarence J. Gamble, November 5, 1947, CGP.
36. Ibid.
37. Roberto Sánchez Vilella, personal interview, June 13, 1978.
38. Clarence J. Gamble, "The Population Experiment of the National Committee on Maternal Health in Puerto Rico," May 19, 1948, p. 1, CGP.
39. Ibid.
40. Deborah C. Leary, Professional Associate, Committee on Human Reproduction, to Clarence J. Gamble, October 14, 1948, CGP.
41. Christopher Tietze to Carmen R. de Alvarado, November 12, 1948, CGP.
42. Christopher Tietze to Robert C. Jones, Pan American Union, December 2, 1948, CGP.
43. *El Mundo*, February 14, 1949.
44. *El Mundo*, February 18, 1949.
45. *El Mundo*, March 8, 1949.
46. Christopher Tietze to Mrs. Carlos V. Torres, June 17, 1949, CGP.
47. Clarence J. Gamble to Wilson Wing, September 10, 1949, CGP.
48. Wilson Wing to Clarence J. Gamble, March 11, 1950, CGP.
49. Ibid.
50. Clarence J. Gamble to Leo Coel, Youngs Rubber Corporation, February 15, 1950, CGP.
51. Wilson Wing to Clarence J. Gamble, March 11, 1950, CGP.
52. Wilson M. Wing, Matthew Tayback, and Clarence J. Gamble, "Birth Control in a Rural Area of Puerto Rico," *Eugenics Quarterly* 5 (1958): 154.
53. Wilson Wing to José S. Belaval, October 9, 1950, CGP.
54. Ibid.
55. Wilson Wing to Clarence J. Gamble, October 20, 1950, CGP.
56. Wilson Wing to Clarence J. Gamble, May 18, 1951, CGP.
57. Wilson Wing to Clarence J. Gamble, July 4, 1953, CGP.
58. Ibid.
59. Clarence J. Gamble to Wilson Wing, July 30, 1953, CGP.
60. Ibid.
61. Clarence J. Gamble to Wilson Wing, October 13, 1953, CGP.
62. Family Planning Association of Puerto Rico, "The Family Planning Program of Puerto Rico" (n.d. [c. 1966]), Puerto Rico Family Planning Association Files, San Juan, Puerto Rico.
63. Wing, Tayback, and Gamble, "Birth Control in a Rural Area," p. 156.
64. Wilson Wing to Clarence J. Gamble, December 23, 1954, CGP.
65. Ibid.
66. Edris Rice-Wray to Clarence J. Gamble, February 23, 1956, CGP.
67. Clarence J. Gamble to Edris Rice-Wray, April 12, 1956, CGP.
68. Wing, Tayback, and Gamble, "Birth Control in a Rural Area," p. 160.
69. "History of the Pathfinder Fund's Involvement in Latin America" (n.d.), CGP.

Chapter 9

1. James Reed, *From Private Vice to Public Virtue* (New York: Basic Books,

1978), p. 340.
2. Ibid.
3. M. C. Chang, "Development of the Oral Contraceptives," *American Journal of Obstetrics and Gynecology* 95 (1978): 217.
4. Ibid.
5. Reed, *From Private Vice*, pp. 332–33.
6. Ibid., p. 340.
7. Ibid., p. 339.
8. Ibid., p. 340.
9. John Rock, quoted in Albert Q. Maisel, *The Hormone Quest* (New York: Random House, 1965), p. 117.
10. Kenneth S. Davis, "The Story of the Pill," *American Heritage* 29 (1978): 85.
11. Maisel, *Hormone Quest*, p. 118.
12. Davis, "Story of the Pill," p. 85.
13. Reed, *From Private Vice*, p. 355.
14. Ibid., p. 354.
15. Davis, "Story of the Pill," p. 85.
16. Maisel, *Hormone Quest*, p. 120.
17. Ibid.
18. Davis, "Story of the Pill," p. 85.
19. Ibid.
20. Maisel, *Hormone Quest*, p. 121.
21. Chang, "Development of the Oral Contraceptives," p. 217; and Maisel, *Hormone Quest*, p. 122.
22. Reed, *From Private Vice*, p. 358.
23. Gregory Pincus to David Tyler, January 14, 1954, and Gregory Pincus to Katherine D. McCormick, March 5, 1954, Gregory Pincus Papers, Library of Congress, Washington, D.C. (hereafter cited as GPP).
24. Gregory Pincus to Katherine D. McCormick, March 5, 1954, GPP.
25. Celso-Ramón García, personal interview, September 16, 1978.
26. Gregory Pincus to Katherine D. McCormick, March 5, 1954, GPP.
27. Gregory Pincus to Margaret Sanger, March 23, 1954, Margaret Sanger Papers, Sophia Smith Collection, Smith College, Northampton, Massachusetts (hereafter cited as MSP).
28. Gregory Pincus to David Tyler, July 21, 1954, GPP.
29. Ibid.
30. Paul Vaughan, *The Pill on Trial* (New York: Coward-McCann, 1970), p. 41.
31. Celso-Ramón García, personal interview, September 16, 1978.
32. Katherine D. McCormick, notes on talk with Dr. Pincus, February 1, 1955, MSP.
33. Ibid.
34. Vaughan, *The Pill on Trial*, p. 39.
35. Gregory Pincus to Katherine D. McCormick, August 26, 1954, GPP.
36. Ibid.
37. Manuel Fernández Fuster to Gregory Pincus, October 12, 1954, GPP.
38. Celso-Ramón García to Gregory Pincus, June 18, 1955, GPP.
39. Procedures for Progesterone Tests, n.d. (c. 1954), GPP.
40. David Tyler to Gregory Pincus, July 8, 1955, GPP.
41. José Díaz Carazo to Gregory Pincus, January 31, 1956, GPP.
42. Chang, "Development of the Oral Contraceptives," pp. 217–18.
43. Davis, "Story of the Pill," p. 86.
44. Solly Zuckerman, *From Apes to Warlords* (New York: Harper and Row, 1978).
45. *London Observer*, January 15, 1956.
46. Davis, "Story of the Pill," p. 86.
47. Katherine D. McCormick, notes from conversation with Dr. Rock, October 6, 1955, MSP.

48. Ibid. In later years, Rock argued that "the pill is simply an 'adjunct to nature' and therefore is not one of the 'unnatural' methods of birth control proscribed by his church." David Hendin, *The Life Givers* (New York: William Morrow, 1976), p. 225. The Catholic church has not accepted this argument.

49. Katherine D. McCormick, notes on conversation with Dr. Rock, January 9, 1956, MSP.

50. Ibid.

51. Ibid.

52. Gregory Pincus to David Tyler, December 30, 1955, GPP.

53. Davis, "Story of the Pill," p. 89.

54. Gregory Pincus to David Tyler, December 30, 1955, GPP.

55. Ibid.

56. Gregory Pincus to David Tyler, July 21, 1954, GPP.

57. Gregory Pincus to Edris Rice-Wray, January 18, 1956, GPP.

58. Ibid.

59. Gregory Pincus to Mr. and Mrs. Edward Hellmick, March 10, 1956, GPP.

60. Katherine D. McCormick, notes on conversation with Dr. Pincus, March 5, 1956, MSP.

61. Edris Rice-Wray to Gregory Pincus, April 17, 1956. GPP.

62. Katherine D. McCormick, notes on conversation with Dr. Pincus, March 5, 1956, MSP.

63. Edris Rice-Wray to Gregory Pincus, April 17, 1956, GPP.

64. Katherine D. McCormick, notes on conversation with Dr. Pincus, March 5, 1956, MSP.

65. Edris Rice-Wray, "Field Study with Enovid as a Contraceptive Agent," Proceedings of a Symposium on 19-Nor Progestational Steroids, Searle Research Laboratories, Chicago, 1957, p. 79.

66. Ibid.

67. Ibid.

68. Edris Rice-Wray to Gregory Pincus, April 17, 1956, GPP.

69. Rice-Wray, "Field Study with Enovid," p. 80; and *El Imparcial*, April 21, 1956.

70. Iris Rodríguez Pla to Gregory Pincus, May 8, 1956, GPP.

71. Ibid.

72. Edris Rice-Wray to Gregory Pincus, June 11, 1956, GPP.

73. Gregory Pincus to Edris Rice-Wray, August 6, 1956, GPP.

74. J. William Crosson, Assistant Director for Clinical Research, Searle, to Edris Rice-Wray, August 27, 1957, Puerto Rico Family Planning Association files, San Juan, Puerto Rico.

75. Vaughan, *The Pill on Trial*, p. 42.

76. Ibid., p. 44.

77. Gregory Pincus to Katherine D. McCormick, October 11, 1956, GPP.

78. Katherine D. McCormick, notes on conversation with Dr. Rock, October 10, 1956, MSP.

79. Edris Rice-Wray to Gregory Pincus, December 20, 1956, GPP.

80. Rice-Wray, "Field Study with Enovid," pp. 81–85.

81. Katherine D. McCormick, notes on conversation with Dr. Pincus, May 16, 1957, MSP.

82. Gregory Pincus to Margaret Sanger, July 22, 1957, MSP.

83. Katherine D. McCormick, notes on conversation with Dr. Pincus, May 16, 1957, MSP.

84. Maisel, *Hormone Quest*, pp. 136–37.

85. Ibid., p. 137.

86. Katherine D. McCormick, notes on conversation with Dr. Pincus, March 5, 1956, and notes on conversation with Dr. Rock, October 10, 1956, MSP.

87. "The Pills," *Time*, February 17, 1961, p. 39.

88. Gregory Pincus to Margaret Sanger, July 22, 1957, MSP.

89. Clarence J. Gamble to Dr. John Smith, Ryder Memorial Hospital, November 8, 1956, Clarence J. Gamble Papers, Countway Library, Boston (hereafter cited as CGP).

90. "History of the Pathfinder Fund's Involvement in Latin America" (n.d.), CGP.

91. Clarence J. Gamble to Margaret Sanger, March 13, 1957, MSP.

92. Doone and Greer Williams, *Every Child a Wanted Child* (Boston: Distributed by Harvard University Press for the Francis A. Countway Library of Medicine, 1978), p. 321.

93. Adaline P. Satterthwaite to Clarence J. Gamble, November 20, 1956, CGP.

94. Adaline P. Satterthwaite to Clarence J. Gamble, July 17, 1957, CGP.

95. Clarence J. Gamble to Adaline P. Satterthwaite, October 18, 1957, CGP.

96. Williams, *Every Child a Wanted Child*, pp. 321–22.

97. J. William Crosson to Clarence J. Gamble, April 2, 1958, CGP.

98. Adaline P. Satterthwaite to Clarence J. Gamble, July 17, 1957, CGP.

99. Adaline P. Satterthwaite to Clarence J. Gamble, December 12, 1957, CGP.

100. Adaline P. Satterthwaite to Clarence J. Gamble, December 2, 1959, CGP.

101. Adaline P. Satterthwaite to Clarence J. Gamble, March 15, 1959, CGP.

102. Ibid.; and Celestina Zalduondo to Clarence J. Gamble, March 30, 1959, CGP.

103. Milton Silverman and Philip R. Lee, *Pills, Profits, and Politics* (Berkeley: University of California Press, 1974), p. 99.

104. J. William Crosson to Clarence J. Gamble, May 4, 1960, CGP.

105. Adaline P. Satterthwaite to Clarence J. Gamble, October 9, 1960, CGP.

106. Adaline P. Satterthwaite to Clarence J. Gamble and accompanying notes on "Field Trial with Norethynodrel, April 1957 to November 1960, Humacao, Puerto Rico," January 13, 1961, CGP.

107. Donald H. Merkin, *Pregnancy as a Disease* (Port Washington, N.Y.: Kennikat Press, 1976), p. 40.

108. Adaline P. Satterthwaite to Clarence J. Gamble, January 26, 1961, CGP.

109. "The Pills," *Time*, February 17, 1961, p. 39.

110. Adaline P. Satterthwaite to Clarence J. Gamble, May 29, 1961, CGP.

111. Clarence J. Gamble to Adaline P. Satterthwaite, June 5, 1961, CGP.

112. Ibid.

113. Adaline P. Satterthwaite to Clarence J. Gamble, July 13, 1961, CGP.

114. Williams, *Every Child a Wanted Child*, p. 326.

115. Clarence J. Gamble to Adaline P. Satterthwaite, June 22, 1962, CGP.

116. Adaline P. Satterthwaite to Clarence J. Gamble, August 25, 1962, CGP.

117. W. M. Jordan, "Pulmonary Em-

bolism," *Lancet* 2 (1961): 1140–41.
118. Silverman and Lee, *Pills, Profits, and Politics*, pp. 98–99.
119. Ibid., p. 99.
120. Adaline P. Satterthwaite to Clarence J. Gamble, August 25, 1962, CGP.
121. Adaline P. Satterthwaite to Clarence J. Gamble, September 12, 1962, CGP.
122. Barbara Seaman and Gideon Seaman, *Women and the Crisis in Sex Hormones* (New York: Bantam Books, 1978), p. 85.
123. Silverman and Lee, *Pills, Profits, and Politics*, p. 99.
124. Adaline P. Satterthwaite to Clarence J. Gamble, September 12, 1962, CGP.
125. "Ryder Memorial Hospital Research Project," March 1, 1963, GPP.
126. Williams, *Every Child a Wanted Child*, p. 327.
127. Lord Platt et al., "Risk of Thromboembolic Disease in Women Taking Oral Contraceptives: Preliminary Report to the Medical Research Council by a Subcommittee," *British Medical Journal* 2 (May 6, 1967): 355, quoted in Silverman and Lee, *Pills, Profits, and Politics*, p. 101.
128. Ibid.
129. "Anticonceptivos Orales," *Population Reports*, Series A(4), April 1978. A recent study, however, found certain types of oral contraceptives to be protective against endometrial cancer. Barbara S. Hulka et al., "Protection Against Endometrial Carcinoma by Combination-Product Oral Contraceptives," *Journal of the American Medical Association* 247 (1982): 475–77.

130. Center for Disease Control, Public Health Service, U.S. Department of Health, Education, and Welfare, "Occupational Exposure to Synthetic Estrogens," *Morbidity and Mortality Weekly Report* 26 (1977): 101.

Chapter 10

1. William B. Breuer, *An American Saga: The Fabulous Tale of Sunnen Products Company* (St. Louis: Pierre Laclede Book, n.d.), p. 79.
2. *The Emko Story*, n.d., p. 3.
3. S. G. Landfather, executive director, Sunnen Foundation, personal communication, November 14, 1978.
4. *The Emko Story*, p. 8.
5. Edris Rice-Wray, personal communication, January 23, 1979.
6. Clarence J. Gamble to Margaret Sanger, August 5, 1956, Margaret Sanger Papers, Sophia Smith Collection, Smith College, Northampton, Massachusetts (hereafter cited as MSP).
7. "Report of the Committee to Develop Plan for the Sunnen Project," August 1956, Clarence J. Gamble Papers, Countway Library, Boston (hereafter cited as CGP).
8. Ibid.
9. Ibid.
10. Ibid.
11. Ibid.
12. Alfred L. Severson to the Puerto Rico Family Planning Association, August 8, 1956, CGP.
13. Family Planning Association of Puerto Rico, "Family Planning Project—Puerto Rico" (n.d. [c. 1964]), Puerto Rico Family Planning Association files, San Juan, Puerto Rico

(hereafter cited as FPA).

14. Wilson M. Wing to Clarence J. Gamble, November 12, 1957, CGP.

15. Nick Thimmesch, "Puerto Rico and Birth Control," *Journal of Marriage and the Family* 30 (1968): 257. The conflict between the mayor of Barceloneta and the Catholic church resulted in the establishment of an alternative church, *Iglesia Católica Antigua*, which followed all Catholic rites and rituals but did not accept the doctrine of the infallibility of the pope. *El Mundo*, October 13, 1961.

16. Press release from the Emko Company, "Data on the Puerto Rican Family Planning Association Program for Mass Distribution of Birth Control Items" (n.d. [c. 1963]), MSP.

17. Ibid.

18. *The Emko Story*, p. 11.

19. Ibid.

20. Ibid.

21. Margaret Sanger Research Bureau, "Report on Single-Dose Test on Aerosol Vaginal Cream #3-J (Sunnen Products)," May 14, 1958; "Report on 21-Day Clinical Test on Aerosol Vaginal Cream, Sunnen Products Co. #33J-4J82," September 11, 1958; "Report on Spermicidal Tests on Aerosol Vaginal Cream #33-J (Sunnen Products)," October 8, 1958, all in FPA.

22. Aquiles J. Sobrero, "Evaluation of a New Contraceptive," *Fertility and Sterility* 11 (1960): 518.

23. Ibid., p. 523.

24. *The Emko Story*, p. 11.

25. Celestina Zalduondo to Clarence J. Gamble, May 20, 1958, CGP.

26. Edris Rice-Wray, personal communication, January 23, 1979.

27. Alfred L. Severson to Celestina Zalduondo, March 21, 1958, CGP.

28. Breuer, *An American Saga*, p. 80.

29. Manuel E. Paniagua, Henry W. Valliant, and Clarence J. Gamble, "Field Trial of a Contraceptive Foam in Puerto Rico," *Journal of the American Medical Association* 177 (1961): 129.

30. Celestina Zalduondo, "Puerto Rico: The Emko Program" report presented to the Third Regional Conference of the International Planned Parenthood Federation, Western Hemisphere Region, Barbados, April 1961.

31. Ibid.

32. Press release from the Emko Company, "Data on the Puerto Rican Family Planning Association Program for Mass Distribution of Birth Control Items" (n.d. [c. 1963]), MSP.

33. Thimmesch, "Puerto Rico and Birth Control," p. 256.

34. Clarence J. Gamble to Matthew Tayback, November 6, 1959, CGP.

35. Press release from the Emko Company, "Data on the Puerto Rican Family Planning Association Program for Mass Distribution of Birth Control Items" (n.d. [c. 1963]), MSP.

36. Ibid.

37. Family Planning Association of Puerto Rico, "Family Planning Project—Puerto Rico" (n.d. [c. 1964]), FPA.

38. S. G. Landfather, personal communication, November 14, 1978.

39. Ibid.

40. Ibid.

41. *The Emko Story*, pp. 15–17.

42. Lazar C. Margulies, "Intrauterine Contraception: A New Approach," *American Journal of Obstetrics and Gynecology* 24 (1964): 515.

43. Adaline P. Satterthwaite to Clarence J. Gamble, October 5, 1961, CGP.
44. Adaline P. Satterthwaite to Clarence J. Gamble, November 23, 1961, CGP.
45. Doone and Greer Williams, *Every Child a Wanted Child* (Boston: Distributed by Harvard University Press for the Francis A. Countway Library of Medicine, 1978), p. 339.
46. Adaline P. Satterthwaite to Clarence J. Gamble, December 14, 1961, and January 8, 1962, CGP.
47. Adaline P. Satterthwaite, "Experience with Oral and Intrauterine Contraception," in Mindel C. Sheps and Jeanne Clare Ridley, eds., *Public Health and Population Change: Current Research Issues* (Pittsburgh: University of Pittsburgh Press, 1965), p. 476.
48. Adaline P. Satterthwaite and Clarence J. Gamble, "Intrauterine Contraception with Plastic Devices Inserted without Cervical Dilation," processed, n.d. (c. 1962), CGP.
49. Adaline P. Satterthwaite, E. Arandes, and M. E. Negrón, "Experience with Intra-uterine Devices in Puerto Rico," in S. J. Segal, A. L. Southam, and K. D. Shafer, eds., *Intrauterine Contraception*, Proceedings of the Second International Conference Sponsored by the Population Council (Amsterdam: Excerpta Medica Foundation, 1964), p. 82.
50. Ibid.
51. William J. Kelly, *A Cost-Effectiveness Study of Clinical Methods of Birth Control: With Special Reference to Puerto Rico* (New York: Praeger, 1972), p. 19.
52. "Approval of Depo-Provera for Contraception Denied," *FDA Bulletin*, March–April 1978, p. 10.
53. "A National Voice for Women's Health Concerns," *Health PAC Bulletin* 11 (1979): 22.
54. *FDA Bulletin*, p. 11.
55. Ibid., p. 10.
56. Ibid.
57. Carol Levine, "Depo-Provera and Contraceptive Risk: A Case Study of Values in Conflict," *Hastings Center Report* 9 (August 1979): 8.
58. Ibid.

Chapter 11

1. "Puerto Rico: The Emko Program," prepared by the Population Council, *Studies in Family Planning*, (1) July 1963, p. 8.
2. The irreversibility of the procedure is presumed throughout the period covered in this account. Recent advances regarding the reversibility of surgical sterilization are discussed in I. Brossens, ed., *Reversibility of Female Sterilization* (New York: Academic Press, 1978). A sterilization plug which may be reversible has been described as a possible "major breakthrough." *Raleigh News and Observer*, November 17, 1981.
3. As indicated in chapter 4, the 1937 legislation governing contraception in Puerto Rico had established a Eugenics Board and authorized the involuntary sterilization of the mentally diseased or retarded, epileptics, and sexual perverts. A total of 97 sterilizations were carried out under this law between 1937 and 1950. *El Mundo*, November 17, 1951.
4. Gilbert W. Beebe and José S. Belaval, "Fertility and Contraception in Puerto Rico," *Puerto Rico Journal of*

Public Health and Tropical Medicine 18 (1942): 34.

5. Ibid., p. 29.

6. J. Mayone Stycos, "Female Sterilization in Puerto Rico," *Eugenics Quarterly* 1 (1954): 3.

7. Charis Gould to Clarence Gamble, July 17, 1941, Clarence J. Gamble Papers, Countway Library, Boston (hereafter cited as CGP).

8. Christopher Tietze to the National Committee on Maternal Health, October 20, 1946, CGP.

9. Christopher Tietze, report #9, September 26, 1946, CGP.

10. Christopher Tietze, report #3, September 19, 1946, CGP.

11. *El Mundo*, February 19, 1945.

12. Christopher Tietze, report #9, September 26, 1946, CGP.

13. Ibid.

14. Ibid.

15. Christopher Tietze to National Committee on Maternal Health, October 20, 1946, CGP. The Health Department's unofficial policy would have met with the approval of President Franklin D. Roosevelt. In 1945 the president discussed the problem posed by Puerto Rico's high birthrate with Charles Taussig, his adviser on Caribbean affairs: "Roosevelt jokingly said: 'I guess the only solution is to use the methods which Hitler used effectively.' He [Roosevelt] said that it is all very simple and painless—'you have people pass through a narrow passage and then there is the brrrrr of an electrical apparatus. They stay there for twenty seconds and from then on they are sterile.'" Quoted from the Charles Taussig Papers, Franklin D. Roosevelt Library, Hyde Park, in William Roger Louis, *Imperialism at Bay: The United States and the Decolonization of the British Empire, 1941–1945* (New York: Oxford University Press, 1978), note on pp. 486–87.

16. Christopher Tietze, report #8, September 25, 1946, CGP.

17. Christopher Tietze, personal interview, June 14, 1979.

18. Christopher Tietze to the National Committee on Maternal Health, October 20, 1946, CGP.

19. Christopher Tietze, report #7, September 24, 1946, CGP.

20. Christopher Tietze, report #2, September 18, 1946, CGP.

21. Ibid.

22. Ibid.

23. Christopher Tietze, report #17, October 7, 1946, CGP.

24. Christopher Tietze, "Human Fertility in Puerto Rico," *American Journal of Sociology* 53 (1947): 40.

25. *El Mundo*, October 21, 1947.

26. *El Mundo*, October 27, 1947.

27. The Puerto Rico Medical Association also stated that the socioeconomic indication for contraception struck down in 1939 as conflicting with federal law could now stand, since the federal legislation had been repealed. Thus the association's legal counsel stressed the broad interpretation that could legitimately be given to the physicians' purview. *El Mundo*, October 17, 1947.

28. Paul K. Hatt, *Backgrounds of Human Fertility in Puerto Rico* (Princeton: Princeton University Press, 1952), pp. 443–44.

29. Ibid., p. 443.

30. Ibid., p. 447.

31. Ibid., p. 450.

32. Quoted in Allan Chase, *The Legacy of Malthus* (New York: Alfred A. Knopf, 1977), p. 371.

33. Unsigned, undated (c. 1947–48), RG 126, box 1137, National Archives.
34. Ibid., p. 11.
35. Ibid., p. 12.
36. Ibid., p. 17.
37. *El Mundo*, February 14, 1949.
38. Stycos, "Female Sterilization," p. 4.
39. *El Mundo*, November 10, 1951.
40. Christopher Tietze, report #4, September 20, 1946, CGP.
41. Harriet B. Presser, *Sterilization and Fertility Decline in Puerto Rico* (Berkeley: Institute of International Studies, University of California, 1973), p. 29.
42. Stycos, "Female Sterilization," p. 4.
43. *El Mundo*, September 7, 1951.
44. *El Mundo*, September 15, 1951.
45. *El Mundo*, September 25, 1951.
46. *El Mundo43*, November 17, 1951.
47. *El Mundo*, October 29, 1952.
48. *El Mundo*, October 31, 1952.
49. *El Mundo*, November 3, 1952.
50. Ibid.
51. José S. Belaval, Emilio Cofresí, and José L. Janer, "Opinión de la Clase Médica de Puerto Rico sobre el Uso de la Esterilización y los Contraceptivos," mimeographed, 1953.
52. Reuben Hill, J. Mayone Stycos, and Kurt W. Back, *The Family and Population Control* (Chapel Hill: University of North Carolina Press, 1959), pp. 166–67.
53. Ibid., pp. 178–79.
54. Ibid., p. 179.
55. Ibid., pp. 179–80.
56. The interaction between contraceptive technology and motivation has been convincingly described as follows: "The technology of modern contraception or abortion may be adopted ... by many of the large number of couples who are not committed to having another pregnancy start as soon as possible after the last delivery. Such behavior can—if it does successfully prevent conception for a while—permit embarking on new, rewarding activities that are conditioned on not being pregnant, and, in turn, reinforce the continuation of fertility regulation and further delaying another pregnancy." Steven Polgar and John F. Marshall, "The Search for Culturally Acceptable Fertility Regulating Methods," in L. H. Hogan and E. E. Hunt, eds., *Health and the Human Condition: Perspectives in Medical Anthropology* (North Scituate, Mass.: Duxbury Press, 1978), p. 339.
57. Hill, Stycos, and Back, *The Family and Population Control*, p. 181.
58. Clarence Senior, "Sterilization in Puerto Rico," in Garrett Hardin, ed., *Population, Evolution and Birth Control* (San Francisco: Freeman, 1964), p. 307.
59. Family Planning Association, "The Family Planning Program of Puerto Rico" (n.d. [c. 1966]), Puerto Rico Family Planning Association files, San Juan, Puerto Rico.
60. Ibid.
61. Ibid. The vasectomy program had to overcome the fear that men undergoing the operation would become impotent or lose their sexual desire: "One of the [Family Planning Association] doctors helped the program by interviewing some of the men and telling them that he himself had been sterilized. When they would not believe him he pulled down his trousers and showed them the scars." Edris Rice-Wray, "Planned Parenthood in Three Cultures" (Paper presented at the Annual Meeting of the Population Associ-

ation of America, Madison, Wisconsin, May 4, 1962), p. 10.

62. Presser, *Sterilization and Fertility Decline*, pp. 30–31.

63. Manuel E. Paniagua et al., "Medical and Psychological Sequelae of Surgical Sterilization of Women," in Lawrence Lader, ed., *Foolproof Birth Control: Male and Female Sterilization* (Boston: Beacon Press, 1972), p. 171.

64. H. C. Barton, "The Employment Situation in Puerto Rico and Migratory Movement between Puerto Rico and the United States," paper presented at a workshop on the employment problems of Puerto Ricans sponsored by the Center for the Study of the Unemployed, Graduate School of Social Work, New York University, May 20–21, 1968, p. 38.

65. By 1960 one-fourth of all U.S. brassieres and electric shavers were manufactured in Puerto Rico. Ralph Hancock, *Puerto Rico: Success Story* (Princeton: Van Nostrand, 1960), p. 164, quoted in Nathan Glazer and Daniel Patrick Moynihan, *Beyond the Melting Pot* (Cambridge: MIT Press, 1963), p. 96.

66. Barton, "The Employment Situation," p. 39.

67. Adaline P. Satterthwaite, "Experience with Oral and Intrauterine Contraception in Rural Puerto Rico," in Mendel C. Sheps and Jeanne Clare Ridley, eds., *Public Health and Population Change: Current Research Issues* (Pittsburgh: University of Pittsburgh Press, 1965), p. 475.

68. Asociación Puertorriqueña Pro Bienestar de la Familia, 1964.

69. Presser, *Sterilization and Fertility Decline*, p. 56.

70. Ibid., p. 175.

71. Ibid., p. 130.

72. Ibid., p. 147.

73. Ibid.

74. Ibid., pp. 55–56.

75. The "voluntariness" of surgical sterilization is discussed in Rosalind Pollack Petchesky, "Reproduction, Ethics, and Public Policy: The Federal Sterilization Regulations," *Hastings Center Report* 9 (1979): 29–41.

76. Leopoldo Figueroa, "Informe Anual del Hospital de Maternidad de San Juan, Año 1933–34," *Boletín de la Asociación Médica de Puerto Rico* 26 (1934): 322.

77. Zoraida Fernández, personal interview, March 6, 1979.

78. Hill, Stycos, and Back, *The Family and Population Control*, p. 171.

79. Roy J. Stokes, "Tubal Ligations," *Boletín de la Asociación Médica de Puerto Rico* 40 (1948): 108.

80. Hill, Stycos, and Back, *The Family and Population Control*, p. 171.

81. *El Mundo*, May 14, 1955.

82. *El Mundo*, December 15, 1958.

83. Ibid.

84. *El Mundo*, December 20, 1958.

85. *El Mundo*, May 2, 1963.

86. The Clergy Consultation Service on Abortion in New York City and comparable groups elsewhere in the United States counseled pregnant women and referred them to Puerto Rico. According to Lader, the clinics to which referrals to Puerto Rico were made were inspected and their services monitored; after physicians began to boost their prices, referrals were mostly made "to one clinic, which maintained superior medical and pricing standards." Lawrence Lader, *Abortion II: Making the Revolution* (Boston: Beacon Press, 1973), p. 46. Other references to

Puerto Rico's role in this abortion network appear in Malcolm Potts, Peter Diggory, and John Peel, *Abortion* (Cambridge: Cambridge University Press, 1977), p. 268; and Bernard N. Nathanson, *Aborting America* (New York: Doubleday, 1979), pp. 23–25, 37–38.

87. *El Mundo*, May 2, 1963.

88. Interestingly, Puerto Rican women were charged less for the same procedure. *El Mundo*, May 4, 1963.

89. Asociación Puertorriqueña Pro Bienestar de la Familia, "¡No matarás!" (n.d.). The FPA's principal sponsor, however, supported abortion. In 1969, Joseph Sunnen participated in a campaign "to demolish the rigidity of hospital abortion practices" in California. After 1970 the Sunnen Foundation assisted the National Association for Repeal of Abortion Laws, the united front which not only spearheaded the liberalization of legislation and the testing of the constitutionality of existing statutes but also promoted a national referral network and alternative service provisions. Lader, *Abortion II*, p. 110.

90. *El Mundo*, May 8, 1963.
91. *El Mundo*, May 30, 1963.
92. *El Mundo*, May 19, 1964.
93. *El Mundo*, November 27, 1967.
94. Ibid.
95. Ibid.
96. Ibid.
97. *San Juan Star*, March 10, 1970.
98. *El Mundo*, April 16, 1970.
99. *El Mundo*, April 27, 1970.
100. *El Mundo*, April 29, 1970.
101. *San Juan Star*, April 19, 1980.

Chapter 12

1. Robert W. Anderson, *Party Politics in Puerto Rico* (Stanford: Stanford University Press, 1965), pp. 111, 215.
2. *San Juan Star*, May 4, 1960.
3. *San Juan Star*, May 23, 1960.
4. *El Mundo*, May 27, 1960.
5. Despite its name, the party's orientation was not broadly Christian but exclusively Catholic. Its symbol was the rosary; its colors, gold and white, those of the Vatican. Religious emblems and references to the Virgin Mary were intertwined with political slogans and canvassing efforts. As a result, prominent Protestant leaders publicly opposed the party and urged their followers to protect the principles of separation of church and state, freedom of conscience, and civil liberty. *San Juan Star*, August 6, 1960.
6. Carlos G. Ramos Bellido, "The Politics of Birth Control in Puerto Rico," Ph.D. diss., University of California at Berkeley, 1977, p. 124.
7. *San Juan Star*, July 6, 1960.
8. *San Juan Star*, July 2, 1960.
9. *San Juan Star*, July 6, 1960.
10. *San Juan Star*, July 22, 1960.
11. *San Juan Star*, July 14, 1960.
12. Quoted in William C. Baggs, "Puerto Rico: Showcase of Development," *1962 Britannica Book of the Year* (Encyclopaedia Britannica, Inc.), p. 23.
13. Ibid., p. 35.
14. *San Juan Star*, October 12, 1960.
15. Ibid., and *San Juan Star*, July 14, 1960.
16. *San Juan Star*, August 15, 1960.
17. *San Juan Star*, October 14, 1960
18. Popular Democratic Party Platform, 1960.

19. Quoted in *New York Times*, October 24, 1960.
20. *San Juan Star*, October 24, 1960.
21. *New York Times*, October 24, 1960.
22. *New York Times*, October 28, 1960.
23. Ibid.
24. *San Juan Star*, October 24, 1960.
25. *San Juan Star*, October 22, 1960.
26. *San Juan Star*, October 25, 1960.
27. *San Juan Star*, October 29, 1960.
28. Ibid.
29. *El Mundo*, October 26, 1960.
30. *El Mundo*, November 2, 1960.
31. *El Mundo*, November 5, 1960.
32. *El Mundo*, November 7, 1960.
33. *New York Times*, October 26, 1960.
34. Quoted in *San Juan Star*, January 29, 1974.
35. *San Juan Star*, November 15, 1960.
36. *San Juan Star*, November 21, 1960.
37. *San Juan Star*, November 23, 1960.
38. Ibid.
39. Rafael Menéndez Ramos, personal interview, December 20, 1978.
40. Celestina Zalduondo to Clarence J. Gamble, October 3, 1962, Clarence J. Gamble Papers, Countway Library, Boston.
41. José Nine Curt, personal interview, April 11, 1978.
42. Ibid.
43. José Nine Curt to Guillermo Arbona, "Summary of Interview with Archbishop, May 15, 1963," May 19, 1963, Nine Curt files.
44. *New York Times*, August 7, 1963.
45. *San Juan Star*, August 7, 1963.
46. *El Mundo*, September 17, 1963.
47. *El Mundo*, October 11, 1963.
48. *New York Times*, August 7, 1963.

Chapter 13

1. Héctor López Pumarejo, "The Prospects for Centralized Comprehensive Planning under Conditions of Dependency: The Puerto Rican Case," Ph.D. diss., Cornell University, 1978, p. 8.
2. José L. Vázquez Calzada, *La Población de Puerto Rico y su Trayectoria Histórica* (Río Piedras: Escuela de Salud Pública, Universidad de Puerto Rico, 1978), p. 276.
3. *San Juan Star*, March 20, 1967.
4. Ernest Gruening, *Many Battles* (New York: Liveright, 1973), p. 485.
5. Quoted in David M. Kennedy, *Birth Control in America* (New Haven: Yale University Press, 1970), p. viii.
6. Gruening, *Many Battles*, pp. 489-90.
7. Ibid.
8. Family Planning Association of Puerto Rico, "The Family Planning Program of Puerto Rico" (n.d. [c. 1966]), Puerto Rico Family Planning Association files, San Juan, Puerto Rico (hereafter cited as FPA).
9. This policy is described in Peta Murray Henderson, "Population Policy, Social Structure and the Health System in Puerto Rico: The Case of Female Sterilization," Ph.D. diss., University of Connecticut, 1976, p. 171.
10. Ibid., and Zoraida Fernández, personal interview, March 6, 1976.
11. Family Planning Association, "The Family Planning Program of

Puerto Rico," FPA.

12. Jean Sharpe, "The Birth Controllers," in Claudia Dreifus, ed., *Seizing Our Bodies* (New York: Vintage Books, 1978), p. 69.

13. *San Juan Star*, August 22, 1968.

14. *San Juan Star*, January 15, 1969.

15. *San Juan Star*, March 20, 1969.

16. Teodoro Moscoso, personal interview, August 23, 1978.

17. Subcomité Asesor de Población, "Informe al Consejo Asesor del Gobernador para el Desarrollo de Programas Gubernamentales" (San Juan: 1969), p. 23.

18. Ibid., p. 17.

19. Ibid., p. 16.

20. Ibid., p. 21.

21. Ibid., p. 27.

22. *San Juan Star*, January 15, 1970.

23. Ibid.

24. *El Imparcial*, January 22, 1970.

25. *El Mundo*, February 6, 1970.

26. Ibid.

27. *San Juan Star*, February 26, 1970.

28. Puerto Rico Department of Health, Office of the Assistant Secretary for Maternal and Child Health Care, "Proposal for Islandwide Family Planning Program," April 1970, p. 7, files of the Puerto Rico Health Department, San Juan, Puerto Rico (hereafter cited as HD).

29. Ibid., p. 10.

30. Dr. José O. Curet to Dr. José Alvarez de Choudens, "Memorandum on the Family Planning Program," January 1973, HD.

31. Subcomité Asesor de Población, "Informe al Consejo Asesor," p. 20.

32. Peter J. Davies, "Trip Report, Puerto Rico, December 5–7, 1973," FPA.

33. Ibid.

34. *El Mundo*, December 3, 1973.

35. Davies, "Trip Report."

36. Herman Nickel, "Puerto Rico's Drift toward Statehood—and Dependence," *Fortune*, August 13, 1979, p. 165.

37. Junta de Planificación, Estado Libre Asociado de Puerto Rico, *Informe Económico al Gobernador*, 1973, p. 11.

38. Junta de Planificación, Estado Libre Asociado de Puerto Rico, *Informe Económico al Gobernador*, 1976, quoted in Vázquez Calzada, *La Población de Puerto Rico*, p. 106.

39. Davies, "Trip Report."

40. Ibid.

41. Ibid.

42. Ibid.

43. "Mensaje del Honorable Gobernador Rafael Hernández Colón a Séptima Asamblea Legislativa en su Segunda Sesión Ordinaria," January 1974.

44. *San Juan Star*, February 7, 1974.

45. Puerto Rico Department of Health, Office of the Assistant Secretary for Maternal and Child Health Care, "Proposal for Islandwide Program," p. 7, HD.

46. *San Juan Star*, February 27, 1974.

47. *San Juan Star*, March 27, 1974.

48. Secretaría Auxiliar de Planificación Familiar, "Plan de Trabajo, 1975–76," September 25, 1974, p. 33, HD.

49. *San Juan Star*, February 27, 1974.

50. *San Juan Star*, April 20, 1974.

51. Rafael Hernández Colón, personal interview, January 12, 1979.

52. Ibid.

53. Antonio Silva Iglecia, personal interview, January 31, 1979.

54. Rafael Hernández Colón, per-

sonal interview, January 12, 1979.

55. Antonio Silva Iglecia, personal interview, January 31, 1979; Departamento de Salud, Secretaría Auxiliar de Planificación Familiar, "Manual de Normas y Procedimientos" (n.d. [c. 1974–75]), appendix A, p. 1, HD.

56. "Informe Anual de la Comisión para el Mejoramiento de los Derechos de la Mujer, julio 1976–junio 1977," December 13, 1977, p. 28.

57. *San Juan Star*, June 11, 1976.

58. Antonio Silva Iglecia, address delivered to the Puerto Rico Public Health Association, San Juan, Puerto Rico, March 25, 1977.

59. *San Juan Star*, June 11, 1976.

60. Departamento de Salud, Programa de Planificación Familiar, "Esterilizaciones Realizadas, Años Fiscales 1974–75, 1975–76, 1976–77, 1977–78," 1980, HD.

61. *San Juan Star*, January 22, 1975.

62. Puerto Rico Department of Health, *Annual Vital Statistics Report, 1977*, 1977, p. 1.

63. *San Juan Star*, September 13, 1968.

64. Puerto Rico Department of Health, "Continuing Application," July 1977–June 1978, p. 1, HD.

65. Sección de Evaluación e Información, División de Programas Categóricos, Secretaría Auxiliar de Servicios Ambulatorios, Departamento de Salud, "Informe Anual, 1978–79: Programa de Planificación de la Familia," November 1979, HD.

66. *San Juan Star*, June 29, 1980.

67. *Nation's Health*, June 1979.

68. *San Juan Star*, June 29, 1980.

69. In addition, the current public policy is oblivious to the weight of historical evidence, which suggests that fertility control "probably cannot be accomplished without heavy reliance on abortion, and the effectiveness of induced abortion—whether legal or illegal—in controlling rapid population growth has been demonstrated on numerous occasions." Malcolm Potts and Pouru Bhiwandiwala, eds., *Birth Control–An International Assessment* (Baltimore: University Park Press, 1979), p. 189.

Chapter 14

1. José L. Vázquez Calzada, *La Población de Puerto Rico y Su Trayectoria Histórica* (Río Piedras: Escuela de Salud Pública, Universidad de Puerto Rico, 1978), p. 171.

2. *Caribbean Business*, September 24, 1980. This represents an annual average of $1,400 per person, substantially in excess of the total per capita income of most of the population of the "developing world."

3. The original estimate of 4 million was based on the number of households; it failed to take into account a significant reduction in the average number of persons per household. *San Juan Star*, May 11, 1980.

4. For example, Argentina, Chile, and Uruguay all have lower crude birthrates than Puerto Rico.

5. Kent C. Earnhardt, "Development Planning and Population Policy in Puerto Rico, 1898–2075: From Historical Evolution to a Plan for Population Stabilization," processed (Río Piedras: Graduate School of Planning, University of Puerto Rico, 1976), p. 138.

6. José L. Vázquez Calzada and Zoraida Morales Del Valle, "Female Sterilization in Puerto Rico and Its

Demographic Effectiveness," processed (Río Piedras: Demography Section, School of Public Health, University of Puerto Rico, 1981).

7. The sterilization rate is based on a survey of ever-married women between the ages of 20 and 49. José L. Vázquez Calzada, "Survey of the Reproductive Cycle of Puerto Rican Women," processed (Río Piedras: Demography Section, School of Public Health, University of Puerto Rico, 1976).

8. "Esterilización M/F," *Population Reports*, October 1978, p. M-12.

9. "Las Encuestas de Prevalencia del Uso de Anticonceptivos: Una Nueva Fuente de Datos Sobre Planificación Familiar," *Population Reports*, October 1981, p. M-8.

10. Ibid.

11. Center for Disease Control, *Morbidity and Mortality Weekly Report*, April 20, 1979, p. 1.

12. William J. Kelly, *A Cost-Effectiveness Study of Clinical Methods of Birth Control: With Special Reference to Puerto Rico* (New York: Praeger, 1972), p. 91.

13. José L. Vázquez Calzada, "La esterilización femenina en Puerto Rico," *Revista de Ciencias Sociales* 18, no. 3 (1973): 294.

14. Vázquez Calzada and Morales del Valle, "Female Sterilization."

15. José L. Vázquez Calzada, "Survey of the Reproductive Cycle."

16. Vázquez Calzada, "La esterilización femenina," p. 306.

17. Department of Health, Commonwealth of Puerto Rico, *Vital Statistics Annual Report: 1980*, August 1981, p. 240.

18. Vázquez Calzada and Morales Del Valle, "Female Sterilization."

19. Several social scientists have observed this phenomenon in a variety of contexts; they have also attempted to explain the rationality of high fertility patterns on other grounds. Examples of the latter include Mahmood Mamdani, *The Myth of Population Control: Family, Caste, and Class in an Indian Village* (New York: Monthly Review Press, 1973); and Jagna Wojcicka Sharff, "Free Enterprise and the Ghetto Family," *Psychology Today* 15, no. 3 (March 1981): 41–48.

20. For example, in a survey undertaken in 1968, women of reproductive age indicated knowledge of five different methods on the average, and more than four-fifths were aware of three or more. Vázquez Calzada, *La Población de Puerto Rico*, pp. 183–84. More recent surveys have indicated an even higher degree of technical sophistication among this population.

21. Bernard Berelson, W. Parker Mauldin, and Sheldon J. Segal, "Population: Current Status and Policy Options," working paper #44, Center for Policy Studies (New York: The Population Council, May 1979), p. 11.

22. This has helped to provoke the formulation and elaboration of a host of often fantastic "explanations" not susceptible to validation. Writing more than twenty-five years ago, Josue de Castro focused on diet as a key variable affecting fertility. Indeed, he used Puerto Rico as proof of his theory that "great changes in birth rates follow . . . radical modifications of diet." De Castro states: "From about the turn of the century the island's birth rate had been fluctuating between 42 and 45 births per thousand, but from 1947 onward it fell progressively, and by 1954 it was below 35. This phenomenon can be explained in large part by

dietary changes introduced in 1947, a result of Puerto Rico's altered political orientation." *The Geopolitics of Hunger* (New York: Monthly Review Press, 1977), pp. 132–33. More recently, Richard A. Easterlin has advanced the thesis that fertility is affected by prospective parents' perceptions of their own affluence compared to that of their parents. Thus couples with high incomes relative to those of their parents tend to have more children than those with low relative incomes. *Birth and Fortune: The Impact of Numbers on Personal Welfare* (New York: Basic Books, 1980).

23. Among examples of the latter, reference can be made to the following: Nicholas J. Demerath, *Birth Control and Foreign Policy: The Alternative to Family Planning* (New York: Harper and Row, 1976); and Mahmood Mamdani, *The Myth of Population Control*. Both these books are based upon experience with family planning activities in India.

24. See, for example, P. T. Bauer, *Equality, the Third World, and Economic Delusion* (Cambridge: Harvard University Press, 1981); Julian L. Simon, *The Ultimate Resource* (Princeton: Princeton University Press, 1981); and Theodore W. Schultz, *Investing in People: The Economics of Population Quality* (Berkeley: University of California Press, 1981).

25. Such, for example, is the characterization that has been made by a leading newspaper commentator, Juan M. García Passalacqua, *San Juan Star*, October 5, 1981.

26. Both La Fortaleza and the resident commissioner's office have issued statements suggesting the possible extent of this out-migration. Estimates of 600,000 to 800,000 Puerto Ricans relocating to the United States "in search of the benefits of citizenship unavailable to them as island residents" have been publicized. *Today Newspaper* (Melbourne, Florida), September 14, 1981.

Index

Abortion, 20–21, 32, 144–48, 172–73, 179, 208 (n. 89); fees for, 145–46, 171, 207 (n. 86), 211 (n. 69); incidence of, 144–46, 171
Agriculture, 5, 12–14, 23–25, 34–36, 38, 48, 59, 61, 74, 76, 82–83
Alvarado, Carmen Rivera de, 53, 99
American Birth Control League, 20, 45
American Cancer Society, 120, 123
Americanization of Puerto Rico, 10–11, 31, 90–91
Aponte Martínez, Luis, 152, 164, 169
Arbona, Guillermo, 126, 154

Back, Kurt, 96, 125, 140–41, 145
Barceloneta, 127, 161, 203 (n. 15)
"Battle of production," 70, 74, 76, 81–82, 90, 92, 97, 100
Belaval, José, 39, 41–42, 44–46, 54, 58, 67, 94, 98, 135, 137, 139
Beverley, James R., 27–29, 46
Birth Control League (San Juan), 28–29
Birth Control League of Puerto Rico (Ponce), 20–22, 49
Birthrate, 20, 23, 41, 52, 59–60, 67, 72, 76, 85, 97, 130, 164, 167, 175, 205 (n. 15), 211 (n. 5), 212 (n. 22)
Bourne, Dorothy, 32, 38–39, 46
Bourne, James, 31–32, 37–39, 41–42, 50
"Brain drain," 76–77

Brazil, 36, 80, 177
Brookings Institution, 23–26, 29, 40, 48, 79, 186 (n. 44)
Byrne, Edwin V., 39–40, 43–44, 49–50

Castañer General Hospital, 135–36
Catholic church, 7, 31–33, 98–99, 126, 160; opposition to birth control, 18, 21, 28, 38–52 passim, 57, 112, 119, 127, 135–37, 139–40, 162–63, 174; participation in electoral politics, 140, 149–158
Catholic Daughters of America, 39, 50
Catholicism, 11, 92, 95, 111, 173
Chang, Min-Chueh, 105–6, 110
Chardón, Carlos, 35, 42
Chardón Plan, 35–37, 41, 77
Christian Action party (CAP), 150–51, 155, 208 (n. 5)
Church-state conflicts, 149–58 passim. *See also* Catholic church
Coffee production, 5, 12–13, 23
Cofresí, Emilio, 95, 145
Columbia University, 39, 95, 119
Commonwealth status, 89–90, 196 (nn. 21, 23)
Comstock laws, 19, 49
Consensual unions, 7, 66
Costa Rica, 36, 79, 81, 177
Cycles of hope and despair, 92–93, 173

215

Davis, James P., 150, 152, 154, 156–58, 160
Dazian Foundation, 113, 124
Department of Health, 32, 51–52, 67, 100–101, 112, 114, 122, 127–28, 145–46, 156, 165, 174, 187 (n. 62); birth control programs in, 56–58, 68, 93, 126, 156–71 passim; maternal services in, 41, 47, 57, 93, 103; sterilizations sponsored by, 136–37, 178
Department of Health, Education, and Welfare, U.S., 167, 170
Department of Social Services, 164–65
Depo-Provera, 132–33
Diffie, Bailey W. and Justine Whitfield, 25–26
District hospitals, 100, 136–37, 139
Dominican Republic, 36, 77–79
Draper, William, 160, 166–67

Economic conditions in Puerto Rico, 5, 13–14, 23, 33–35, 40, 43, 55, 59, 72, 159, 166–67, 181
Eisenhower, Dwight D., 160, 166
Emigration, 25, 31, 33, 35–36, 69, 74–82, 85–88, 90, 92–93, 95, 130, 159, 174, 181, 186 (n. 42), 213 (n. 26)
Emigration Advisory Committee, 79–80
Emko foam, 128–131, 134
Employment, 24, 59, 71, 83, 142; of women, 59, 86–87, 142–43
Enovid, 115–22
Estrogen, 106–7, 115, 123
Eugenics, 65, 138–39, 144; as argument against birth control, 27, 33, 66; as rationale for birth control, 20, 38, 41, 48, 51, 163
Eugenics Board, 49, 204 (n. 3)

Family Planning Association of Puerto Rico (Asociación Puertorriqueña pro Bienestar de la Familia), 102–3, 112–13, 121–22, 124–30, 134, 141, 143, 146, 154, 156, 160–62, 164–68, 178
Federal Emergency Relief Administration (FERA), 31, 41–42
Federal legislation, 38, 52, 55, 58–59, 161–62
Fernós Isern, Antonio, 66–68, 79–80, 97
Ferré, Luis A., 151, 162–65, 168, 174
Fertility, 25, 33–34, 41, 48, 95, 104, 138, 174–76, 212 (nn. 19, 22)
Five-hundred acre law, 9, 25, 61–62
Fomento, 65, 67, 70, 71, 74, 76, 80, 83, 86, 94, 142–43, 159, 166
Food and Drug Administration, U.S., 119, 123, 133
Ford Foundation, 123, 163, 174
Free Hospital for Women (Boston), 107, 110, 112

Gamble, Clarence J., 45–47, 50, 53–54, 94, 96, 97, 99, 101–4, 117–18, 121, 125, 129
García, Celso-Ramón, 109–10, 118, 120
Garrido Morales, Eduardo, 52, 57–58, 66–67
Gaylord, Gladys, 39, 42, 45
G. D. Searle Company, 106, 110, 112–13, 115, 118–19
Gore, Robert H., 30–32
Gruening, Ernest, 37, 39, 42–44, 46, 50, 52, 54, 58, 163
Guttmacher, Alan, 119–20

Harvard University, 37, 91, 106, 118, 120
Hatt, Paul, 95, 137, 141, 145
Hayes, Patrick J., 37, 44

Health centers, 126–27
Health conditions in Puerto Rico, 7–8, 10, 24, 26, 28, 43, 55, 84, 86, 94
Health Department. *See* Department of Health
Hernández Colón, Rafael, 166–67, 169–70, 174
Hill, Reuben, 96, 125, 140–42
Hookworm, 8, 10, 24
Hurricanes, 12, 23, 30

Ickes, Harold, 33, 58, 62
Immigration, 34, 159, 170
India, 18–19, 117, 138, 213 (n. 23)
Industrial Development Company, 64–65. *See also* Fomento
Industrialization, 34–35, 40, 69, 71, 73–74, 85, 159
Infant mortality, 8, 17, 22, 84, 92, 163, 180
Informed consent, 117, 137, 169
International Planned Parenthood Federation, 111, 133, 167
Intrauterine devices, 131–32

Jíbaro, 7, 20, 40, 61
Johns Hopkins University, 100–101
Jones Act, 9, 98, 184 (n. 19)

Kennedy, John F., 152–53, 161

Lanauze Rolón, José, 20–22, 29, 185 (n. 28)
Land tenure in Puerto Rico, 9, 12, 14, 24, 26, 35, 48, 60–61
Legislation governing birth control, 9, 22, 28, 49–55, 136, 139, 150, 154, 161, 185 (n. 10), 204 (n. 3), 205 (n. 27)
"Local option," 126, 156

McCormick, Katherine Dexter, 106–9, 111, 113, 124

Machismo, 7, 144, 178
McManus, James E., 150, 152, 155, 160
Malaria, 8, 24, 32, 84, 86, 145
Malthusianism, 16–19, 21
Margaret Sanger Research Bureau, 105, 128
Maternal and Child Health Association (Asociación pro Salud Maternal e Infantil de Puerto Rico), 46–56, 58, 67, 94, 99, 117, 134
Medical profession, 20, 22, 23, 27, 137–38, 140, 145–47. *See also* Puerto Rico Medical Association
Menéndez Ramos, Rafael, 35, 50–51
Midwives, 57, 145, 191 (n. 5)
Mortality, 23–24, 59, 72, 84–85, 92
Moscoso, Teodoro, 70–71, 79–80, 162–63, 166–67, 191 (n. 9)
Mundo, El, 17, 20, 27, 72, 99, 163
Municipal government, 127, 129, 136
Muñoz Marín, Luis, 20, 29, 72, 79, 88, 91, 100, 140, 159, 163; in 1960 elections, 149, 151–56; political career, 60–65, 99; views on birth control, 16–19, 35, 97–98, 126, 166; views on political status of Puerto Rico, 72–74, 139

Naranjito project, 97, 99–101
National Catholic Welfare Conference, 38, 40, 50
National Committee on Maternal Health, 94, 98–99
Nationalist party, 26, 31, 40
Needlework industry, 59, 87, 142
Neo-Malthusianism, 21–22, 114, 136, 150, 181
New Deal, 31, 58, 61, 64, 73, 88
New Progressive party (NPP), 162, 166, 170
New York Times, 37, 79, 157–58
Nine Curt, José, 156–57

Norethindrone, 111–12, 121
Norethynodrel, 111–12, 115

Operación, la, 136, 140–41, 144, 161, 169, 177. *See also* Sterilization
Operation Bootstrap, 82, 85, 87–89, 91–92, 123, 159, 166, 196 (n. 20)
Oral contraception, 103, 104, 109–23 passim, 132, 134; as protective of cancer, 120–21, 123; clinical trials of, 107–23; side effects of, 114–16, 118, 120, 122–23
Ortega, Jacinto, 16, 35
Overpopulation, 13–14, 17, 40, 65

Page, Phyllis, 45–46
Paniagua, Manuel, 116, 120
Party politics in Puerto Rico, 10, 38, 41, 60–63, 140, 149–55, 162, 166, 170
Pastoral letters, 136, 150, 152, 154
Petrochemical industry, 159, 166
"Pill." *See* Oral contraception
Pincus, Gregory, 105–13, 115, 117, 119–21, 123, 125
Planned Parenthood Federation of America, 105, 107, 142
Political status of Puerto Rico, 8–9, 31, 89–91, 181
Pons, Juan A., 98–100, 114–15, 126, 138–39
Popular Democratic party (PDP), 61–62, 72, 74, 81, 98, 139–40, 149–56, 160, 162–63, 166
Population Association (Asociación de Estudios Poblacionales), 94–95, 102, 126, 141
Population Council, 132, 179
Population Crisis Committee, 166–67, 174
Population growth, 5, 23, 59, 93, 175
Population of Puerto Rico, 13–14, 23, 30, 86, 159, 176
Population-resources issue, 17, 24, 28, 34–35, 60, 66–67, 72, 74, 100
Pregnancy rate, 48, 129
Presbyterian Hospital, 27, 47, 135–37
Presser, Harriet, 143–44
Progesterone, 106–12
Protestant: churches, 11, 183 (n. 11); hospitals, 11, 47–48; leaders, 208 (n. 5)
Public Health Service, U.S., 52, 68
Puerto Rican Independence party (PIP), 139, 149–50
Puerto Rico Emergency Relief Administration (PRERA), 31–33, 37–42, 132, 145
Puerto Rico Medical Association, 41, 49, 122, 146–47, 205 (n. 27)
Puerto Rico Planning Board, 64, 67
Puerto Rico Public Health Association, 74, 94, 99
Puerto Rico Reconstruction Administration (PRRA), 42–44, 46, 48, 53, 70, 126, 134

"Red scare," 49, 155
Rhoads, Cornelius, 27
Rhythm method, 42, 102, 154, 157–58, 162
Rice-Wray, Edris, 103, 112–16, 125
Rock, John, 106–9, 111–13, 115, 117, 200 (n. 48)
Rockefeller Foundation, 10, 27
Rodríguez, Iris, 113–15
Rodríguez, Noemí, 118–19
Roosevelt, Eleanor, 32–33, 68
Roosevelt, Franklin D., 30, 34–35, 38, 43, 50, 58–59, 64, 77, 205 (n. 15)
Ryder Memorial Hospital, 47, 117–18, 120–23, 132

Sanger, Margaret, 16–17, 20–22, 26, 29, 37, 50, 105–6, 108, 185 (nn. 18, 19), 187 (n. 62)
Satterthwaite, Adaline P., 117–23, 132
School of Tropical Medicine, 39, 42, 46

Senior, Clarence, 76, 79, 93, 95
Sex: in marriage, 21–22; roles, 7, 142–44; taboos, 141
Side effects: of Depo-Provera, 133; of intrauterine devices, 132; of oral contraceptives, 114–16, 118, 120, 122–23
Silva Iglecia, Antonio, 168–69
Social classes in Puerto Rico, 6, 12–13, 87, 179
Social Science Research Center, 95, 103, 125
Social Security Act, 58, 162
Spanish-American War, 3, 8
Spellman, Francis, 152–53
Statehood Republican party (SRP), 150–51, 155, 162
Sterilization, 42, 100, 114–17, 125, 127, 134–44, 151, 154, 161, 164, 168–69, 171, 176–79, 204 (nn. 2, 3), 207 (n. 75); differences by class, 137, 141, 143–44, 178–79; of minors, 169–70; prevalence, 102, 134–46 passim, 168, 176, 212 (n. 7); regrets over, 138, 179
Stone, Abraham, 105, 128
Stycos, J. Mayone, 96, 125, 139–41, 145
Sugar cane, 5–6, 9, 12, 23, 28, 76
Sugar industry, 12, 24, 26, 34–35, 60, 186 (n. 44); involvement in birth control, 48, 53
Sunnen, Joseph, 124–26, 128–31, 208 (n. 89)
Sunnen Foundation, 125, 130–31, 142, 161
Syntex, 111–12, 121

Tennessee Valley Authority (TVA), 82, 88
Tietze, Christopher, 94, 96–100, 136–37, 139

Tobacco, 5, 12–13, 184 (n. 24)
Torres, Estella Alcaide de, 28, 46, 50, 53–54, 100
Tourism, 83, 88
Trujillo, Rafael Leonidas, 77–78
Trujillo Alto project, 101–4
Tuberculosis, 7, 10, 24, 32, 55, 84, 138
Tugwell, Rexford G., 33–35, 62–66, 73, 77–78
Tyler, David, 108–10, 112, 122

Unemployment, 23–25, 35, 43, 51, 64, 68, 71, 76, 86, 93, 159, 163, 166, 168, 181
Union for the Defense of Natural Morality, 139–40
United States–Puerto Rico relationship, 8–9, 11–12, 14, 52, 60–61, 64, 72–73, 79, 89, 91–92, 98, 167, 170, 174–75, 181
University of Puerto Rico, 32–33, 35, 46, 78, 95, 97, 103, 108, 122, 133
University of Puerto Rico School of Medicine, 108–10, 113, 119, 123, 156–57

Vasectomy, 136, 138, 141, 168, 178, 206 (n. 61)
Venereal disease, 10, 28, 184 (n. 15)
Venezuela, 36, 79, 167

Willinger, Aloysius J., 28, 38, 40
Wing, Wilson, 100–103
Winship, Blanton, 49–50, 58, 62
Worcester Foundation for Experimental Biology, 103, 105–6, 108–9, 113, 116, 118
World War II, 60, 63–64, 68–71, 73–74, 88, 108

Zalduondo, Celestina, 126, 128–30, 145

www.ingramcontent.com/pod-product-compliance
Lightning Source LLC
Chambersburg PA
CBHW021403290426
44108CB00010B/364